INTERMITTENT FASTING FOR WOMEN OVER 50

THE ULTIMATE STEP-BY-STEP GUIDE FOR SENIOR
WOMEN TO LOSE WEIGHT AND INCREASE ENERGY
THROUGH METABOLIC AUTOPHAGY

Table of Content

INTRODUCTION

There are so many strategies for losing weight. How do you know where to start? Women have different needs than men when it comes to dieting, exercise, and weight loss, and it seems that many popular strategies are aimed at men who want to look like muscular bodybuilders. Many of these programs leave you hungry, unsatisfied, and ultimately lead you to quit early without ever seeing results.

Intermittent fasting is a natural way to make you feel and look better, especially when you are in yours 50s. Your body was designed to eat in this way and has been confused by the never-ending availability of food and snacks. This form of patterned eating will restore your energy levels, retain your needed body muscle while reducing body fat, and improve your overall health and wellness. The major problem with traditional diets is that they are just hard to stick to. You deny yourself your favorite food and snacks in hopes of weight loss and when you slip up, you feel ashamed and guilty—resulting in the derailment of your entire routine.

Cycling your eating pattern through periods of eating and fasting is as natural to your body as breathing. Humans have been eating this way for thousands of years, and only recently have we muddled our hunger signals so significantly that they are working against us instead of for us. Allowing yourself unrestricted access to food and snacks day in and day out alters your body's chemistry, increasing the production of hunger-signaling hormones. These hormones now tell your body constantly that you are hungry, and they are hard to ignore! Intermittent fasting will reprogram these hormones, decreasing your hunger signals and resigning them to the proper times of the day.

Changing the way you eat is difficult. By denying yourself your favorite meals, you are setting yourself up for failure. Intermittent fasting allows you to enjoy your favorite foods, snacks, and drinks as long as you are consuming them within your non-fasting window. Limiting the time you have available to consume calories will limit the total number of calories you'll ultimately consume—providing weight loss with little effort. Fasting for weight loss is different than a religious fast or fasting before a medical procedure. It does not mean you don't eat anything and wait for the pounds to fall off. You simply limit your total caloric intake during specific periods of time (hours of the day or days of the week, depending on which method of intermittent fasting you feel is most appropriate for you) while enjoying a normal diet and lifestyle the rest of the time! Reducing the amount of food you eat for short periods of time is simpler and easier to stick to for most women, resulting in success and dedication—without throwing in the towel.

The longer you practice intermittent fasting cycles, the easier you'll find them to be. Your body will adjust, you'll feel more motivation and energy, and you'll wonder how you could have possibly eaten the quantity of food you used to—all day long! This guide will explain in simple terms the science behind intermittent fasting, the benefits you can expect, and how to implement the plan into your life.

CHAPTER 1

WHAT IS
INTERMITTENT FASTING?

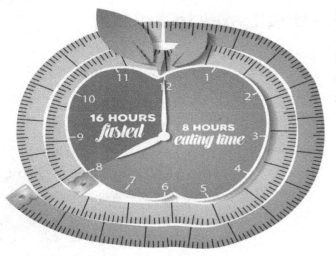

Most individuals know intermittent fasting as losing weight assistance. Intermittent fasting is a lifestyle that allows people to consume fewer calories, leading to weight loss over time.

Without being on an insane diet or consuming the calories to nil, it's a perfect way to get healthy. Most of the time, when one begins intermittent fasting, they'll aim to maintain their calories the same as during a shortened time; most people consume larger meals. In comparison, prolonged fasting is a healthy way to preserve body mass while becoming lean. But most notably, intermittent fasting is among the most beneficial way to be in shape with many other benefits. This is an easy way to get the desired results. If performed properly, intermittent fasting will have valuable advantages, like weight reduction, type 2 diabetes reversal, and several other aspects. Plus, this will save time and resources for you.

Intermittent fasting is successful because it makes it possible for the amount of insulin and blood sugar to reach a low level. The body's fat-storing enzyme is insulin. Fat moves into the fat cells and gets absorbed when insulin levels are high in the blood; if insulin level is low, fat will move and burn out of fat cells. In short, IF is when food is readily available, but you prefer not to consume it. This may be over any period of time, from several hours to a couple of days, or sometimes a week or more under strict medical monitoring. You can begin fasting at any moment of your choice, and you can also end a fast at your will.

You fast intermittently if you don't consume food by choice. For instance, between dinner and breakfast, till the following day, you will not eat and fast for around 12 to 14 hours. Intermittent fasting can, in that way, be deemed a part of daily life.

1. The Science Behind It

Like any idea of eating that quickly takes over health and diet cultures, intermittent fasting has been suspected to be a fad. Still, the evidence behind fasting's advantages is already clear—and increasing.

There are several hypotheses as to why this eating pattern works so well, but tension has to do with the most widely studied—and most proven gain.

The term stress has been vilified continuously, but the body profits from some stress. Exercise, for example, is technically stress on the body (especially on the muscles and the cardiovascular system). Still, this specific stress ultimately makes the body better as long as you implement the correct amount of recovery period into your exercise plan.

Intermittent fasting stresses the body in the same way that exercise does; it brings the cells under moderate tension as you refuse the body food for a certain period. Cells respond to this tension over time by studying the best way to cope with it. It has an improved ability to resist illness because the body becomes better at dealing with pain.

2. The Best Intermittent Fasting Types to Follow

There are so many different ways to practice it. I will guide you through 10 specific and different methods for IF before finishing with a section on how to make your choice. At the end of this chapter, if you have chosen to try the IF, you should feel that your IF plans have direction and form, and you should be excited to implement these new plans in your daily routine.

Explanation of Different Methods

Before you can start and incorporate it into your lifestyle, you must know all the possibilities to choose the right one for you, your goals, your habits, and your body/personality type. Read the following ten tips to discover which methods seem most appropriate.

Lean Gain Method

The method of lean gain essentially focuses on the combined efforts of rigorous exercise, fasting, and a healthy diet. The fame surrounding this approach comes from its acclaimed success in converting fat directly into the muscle. The goal is to fast every day for 14–16 hours, starting from the waking up. The ideal approach to lean gains seems to be to get up and fast until 1:00 pm, stretch, and warm-up before training just before noon. Starting at noon, you would start training in any exercise you choose for an hour or less, and you will end up breaking quickly around 1 pm. Your meal at this time would be the best of the day. You attended your days as always in the past and, as far as possible, return to eat around 4 pm, and then eat for the last time around 9 pm. If you choose this approach and feel a little overwhelmed, you can work up to 15 hours, starting with 13 or 14 hours of fasting only during the first week.

Method 16:8

The 16:8 method is one of the most popular among the fasters. You spend 16 hours on an empty stomach every day, and the other 8 hours are your window to eat. Many people try to choose the 8-hour feeding period as the time when they are most active. If you are a night person, do not hesitate to do it a little later. Stop eating during the day as much as possible and then have breakfast around 3 or 4 in the afternoon. For people who have breakfast early in the morning, for example, around 11 a.m., or lunch from 7 p.m. to 4 a.m. It is an incredibly flexible method that works for many different types of people. It is also flexible when you decide to try a particular fast food relationship. For example, if you don't seem to be playing with the food window from 11 a.m. to 7 p.m., you can change the next day to meet your needs better. You can try to wait until later for breakfast! Try what you need to do, as long as you keep that ratio of 16:8 hours. While the lean gain method technically applies the same hourly rate, it is much more rigorous than a healthy diet and exercise regime. The 16:8 method does not need any exercise reinforcement, but it depends on the professional. It is always better to try to add healthy dietary options to your IF feeding schedule, but do not try to limit too many calories, as it may cause dizziness and low energy. With this method, you can eat what you need and exchange the hours you want.

Method 14:10

Similar to method 16:8, 14:10 requires fasting and feeding on multiple levels every day. In this case, I would fast for 14 hours and then eat for 10 hours. This method has the same flexibility of 16:8 in terms of what time of day it is organized and how easy it is to solve problems. But it is also flexible in the sense that the window for eating lasts two hours longer, it can accommodate people with more intense physical routines or daily needs, as well as people who need to eat a little later during the day.

Method 20:4

While the 14:10 method was a simpler step than the 16:8 method, the 20:4 method is a step forward in terms of difficulty. Without a doubt, it is a more intense method, since it requires 20 hours of fasting every day with only a 4-hour feeding period for the individual to obtain all their nutrients and energy. Many people who try this method end up eating a large meal with several snacks or two smaller meals with fewer snacks. The 20:4 method is flexible in the sense where the individual chooses how the window for eating is divided between meals and snacks.

The 20:4 method is complicated since many people instinctively eat excessively during the feeding window, but it is neither necessary nor healthy. People who choose the 20:4 method should try to keep portions of food the same size they normally would without fasting. Experiencing how many snacks are needed will also be useful in this method. Many people end up working up to 20:4 with other methods, depending on what their bodies are capable of handling and what they are ready to try. Few people begin with 20:4, so if it doesn't work right away, don't be too hard on yourself! Return to 16:8 and then see how soon you can return to where you want to be.

The Warrior Method

The warrior's method is quite similar to the 20:4 method in which the individual fasts for 20 hours a day and stops quickly for a period of 4 hours to eat. However, the difference lies in the perspective and mentality of the professional. The thought process behind the warrior's method is that in ancient times, the hunter who returned home from stalking prey or the warrior who returned home from the battle only received one meal a day.

A meal should provide sustenance for the rest of the day, recovering energy for the future. Therefore, the warrior method professionals are advised to eat an excellent meal when they have breakfast and that the meal should be rich in fat, protein, and carbohydrates for the rest of the day (and for the days to come). However, as with the 20:4 method, it can sometimes be too intense for professionals, and it is very easy to reduce it a lot by inventing a method like 18:6 or 17:7. If it doesn't work, don't force it, but try to do it for a week to see if the problem is your stubbornness or if it is just a coincidence with the method.

12:12 Method

The 12:12 method is somewhat simpler, along with the lines of 14:10, instead of 16:8 or 20:4. Beginners in intermittent fasting would do well to try it immediately. Some people sleep 12 hours every night and can easily wake up from the fasting period, ready to join the window to eat. Many people use this method in their lives without even knowing it. However, to follow the 12:12 method in your life, you will want to be as determined as possible. Be sure to be strict with the limits of 12 hours. Make sure it works and feels good in your body, so we invite you to improve things and try, for example, 14:10 or maybe your invention, like 15:11. As always, start with what works and then go up (or down) to what makes you feel good (and maybe even better).

5:2 Method

The 5:2 method is popular among those who wish to improve things in general. Instead of fasting and eating every day, these people practice fasting two full days a week. The other five days are free to eat, exercise, or diet, but the other two days (which can be consecutive or scattered during the week) must be strictly fasting days. However, for those fasting days, it is not as if the individual cannot eat anything at all. It is allowed to consume no more than 500 calories per day for this intermittent fasting method. I suppose that these days of fasting would be better known as "limited hiring" days, as it is a more precise description. The 5:2 method is extremely rewarding, but it is also one of the most difficult to try. If you have problems with this method, do not be afraid to experiment next week with a method like 14:10 or 16:8, where you fast and eat every day. If this works best for you, stick with it! However, if you have "active" days and "free" days with fasting and feeding, there are also other alternatives.

Eat-Stop-Eat Method (24 Hours)

The method to stop eating for 24 hours is another option for people who want to have "on" and "free" days between fasting and eating. It is a little less intense than the 5:2 method and is much more flexible for the individual, depending on what he needs. For example, if you need a 24-hour literal fast every week and that's it, you can do it. On the other hand, if you want something more flexible than the type of 5:2 method to happen, you can work with what you want and create a method that surrounds those desires and goals. The most successful approaches to the Eat-Stop-Eat method involved a more rigorous diet (or at least a prudent and healthy diet) during the 5 or 6 days in which the individual participates in the free meal window of the week. For the individual to see success with weight loss, there will also have to be a caloric restriction (or a high nutrition approach) those 5 or 6 days, so that the body has a version of consistency in the health and nutrition content. In the one or two days a week that the individual decides to fast, there may still be a very limited calorie intake. As with the 5:2 method, during these fasting days, you cannot consume more than 500 calories in food and beverages so that the body can maintain the flow of energy and more.

If the individual exercises, those training days must be reserved for the 5 or 6 days of free food. The same applies to method 5:2. Try not to exercise (at least not in excess) on the days chosen to fast. Your body will not appreciate the additional stress when you eat so few calories. As always, you can choose to switch from the Eat-Stop-Eat method to another if it works easily and you are interested in something else. Also, you can start with a rigorous 24-hour method and then move on to a more flexible Eat-Stop-Eat approach. Do what you think is right and never be afraid to solve one method simply by choosing another.

Alternate-Day Method

This method is similar to the Eat-Stop-Eat and 5:2 method because it focuses on individual "on" and "off" days for fasting and eating. The difference for this method, in particular, is that you end up fasting at least 2 days a week and sometimes for 4 days. Some people follow very rigorous approaches to the alternate-day method and fast every other day, consuming only 500 calories or less on fasting days. Some people, on the other hand, are much more flexible and tend to eat for two days, one day on an empty stomach, two days, one day on an empty stomach, and so on. This method is even more flexible than getting up in that sense, since it allows the individual to choose how to alternate food and fasting, depending on what works best for the body and mind. The alternate-day method is like a step up from the Eat-Stop-Eat and 24-hour methods, especially if the individual alternates the fast of one day and the next day eating, and so on. Surprisingly, this more intense style of fasting works particularly well for people who work in equally intense fitness regimes. People who consume more calories per day than 2000 (which is true for many bodybuilders and exercise enthusiasts) will have more to gain from this method since they only need to reduce their fasting diet to about 25 percent of the standard caloric intake. Therefore, those fasting days can still provide solid nutritional support to fitness experts, helping them sculpt their bodies and maintain a new level of health.

Spontaneous Omission Method

The alternate-day method and the Eat-Stop-Eat method are certainly flexible in their approaches to when the individual fasts and when he eats. However, none of the plans mentioned above are as flexible as the method of spontaneous omission.

The spontaneous jump method requires the individual to skip meals within each day, whenever you want (and when it is perceived that the body can handle it). Many people with sensitive digestive systems or who practice regimens of more intense physical conditioning will start their experience with IF through the spontaneous jump method before moving on to something more intense. People who have very messy daily schedules or people who are around food a lot but forget to eat will benefit from this method, as it works well with chaotic schedules and unplanned energies. Despite this chaotic and disorganized potential, the method of spontaneous omission can also be more structured and organized, depending on what you do about it! For example, someone who wants more structure can choose which food they want to skip each day. Suppose you choose to skip breakfast every day. Therefore, your method of spontaneous omission will be structured around you, making sure to skip breakfast (that is, do not eat at least until 12:00 p.m.) every day. Whatever you need to do to make this method work, try it! This method is made for experimentation and adventure.

Crescendo Method

The last method that is worth mentioning is the crescendo method, which is very suitable for women to practice (since high-intensity fasts can be very harmful to their anatomy). This approach is made for internal awareness, soft introductions, and gradual additions, depending on what works and what doesn't. It is a very active type of trial and error method. Through the crescendo method, the individual begins to fast only 2 or 3 days a week, and on those days of fasting, it would not be a very intense fast. It would not even be so strict that the individual should not consume more than 500 calories, as with 5:2, Eat-Stop-Eat, and other methods. Instead, these "fast" days would be trial periods for methods such as 12:12, 14:10, 16:8, or 20:4. The remaining 4 or 5 days of the week would be open periods for eating. The professional is encouraged to maintain a healthy diet throughout the week. The crescendo method works extremely well for female practitioners because it allows them to see how methods like 14:10 or 12:12 will affect their bodies without attaching them to the hook, line, and plumb line of the method. It allows them to see what each method does at the hormonal level, menstrual tendency, and mood swings. Therefore, the crescendo method encourages these people to be more in touch with their bodies before moving too fast towards something that can cause serious anatomical and hormonal damage. The crescendo method will also work very well for overweight or diabetic professionals, as it will allow them to have these same "trial period" moments with everyone.

CHAPTER 2

WHY START INTERMITTENT FASTING AT AGE 50?

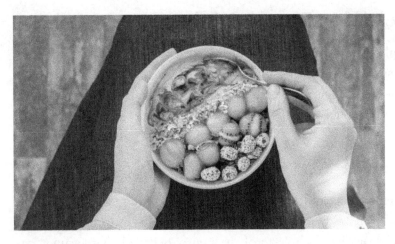

Being a woman is one thing. Being a woman over the age of 50 is another. With age, your body will begin to experience some changes. If you are self-aware, you will notice these changes early and can start work on ways to combat changes that interfere with your health.

At age 50 and over, it also naturally becomes more challenging to lose weight. This is because your metabolism will slow down, joints might be more prone to ache, muscle mass will decrease, and you might even experience sleep issues. In addition to these, you'll become more at risk of developing certain age-related diseases and health conditions.

Some of the changes in your body might be subtle, but they are veiled threats to a fully functional body system and definitely to the longevity we all seek.

This is why it is imperative to seek out measures, lifestyles, and diets that could help you lose fat, especially dangerous belly fat. Losing fat will drastically reduce the risks of developing health issues, such as diabetes, heart attack, and cancer.

Below are a few reasons you need to consider that relate to intermittent fasting:

3. Weight Loss

The most well-known and desirable advantage of intermittent fasting is weight loss. This is understandable; this may also be the main reason why you approached it in the first place. Yet, you may want to explore the topic since there are a lot more advantages that you may not be aware of.

4. Defective Cell Cleaning

Intermittent fasting promotes autophagy, which is how the body disposes of cells that are more likely to get contaminated or become destructive. Faulty cells not working at the highest level can accelerate aging, as well as Alzheimer's disease and type 2 diabetes.

The repairing procedure can be increased during intermittent fasting, as the body does not need to concentrate on food assimilation. Instead, it can completely focus on cell repair. This procedure is called autophagy.

5. Breast Cancer Recurrence Prevention

A more extended time of fasting is another technique used to decrease cancer growth recurrence in breast tissue. A research study with breast cancer survivors found that the women who fasted for longer than 13 hours per night had a significant 36% lower chance of recurrence than the women who fasted for less than 13 hours per night.

6. Lower Risk of Developing Type 2 Diabetes

Type 2 diabetes frequently occurs in people over the age of 45. It can occur when your cells do not react properly to insulin. Insulin is a hormone secreted in the intestine by the pancreas, which permits cells to assimilate and utilize glucose (sugar) as energy. An impressive number of studies have shown a reduction of insulin resistance in patients that follow an intermittent fasting diet. It is best to consult with your doctor if this is applicable to you.

7. Improved Heart Health

Fasting can reduce your resting heart rate, cholesterol levels, and triglycerides. Fasting and better heart health may likewise be connected to how your body processes cholesterol and sugar. Ordinary fasting can diminish your low-density lipoprotein or "bad" cholesterol. It is also believed that fasting may improve how your body processes sugar. This can decrease your danger of putting on weight and help to treat diabetes, which are both risk factors for heart disease.

8. Self-Healing

Intermittent fasting is also a great time for your body to run "self-healing" operations. When you are continually eating, you are not giving your body and your cells the time they need to rest. They need this time to repair themselves or dispose of those cells that may get tainted or destructive. This procedure is called autophagy and can be triggered under specific intermittent fasting conditions.

9. Anti-Aging Process

The modern-day lifestyle includes too much stress and is too passive. Whether we like it or not, these factors contribute to the aging process. You are probably wondering what intermittent fasting can do to slow down this process, or if that is even possible. Intermittent fasting is not "the fountain of youth," and it will not grant you immortality. However, it can still lower your blood pressure and reduce oxidative damage, enhance your insulin sensitivity, and reduce your fat mass. These will all make you feel and look younger, fresher, and extend life expectancy.

10. Therapeutic Benefits

When it comes to therapeutic benefits, the most important ones are physical, spiritual, and psychological. In terms of physical benefits, it can be a powerful cure for diabetes and heart-related issues. It can also prove to be very useful for reducing seizure-related brain damage and seizures themselves and improving the symptoms of arthritis. This practice also has a spiritual value, as it's widely practiced for religious purposes worldwide. Although fasting is regarded as penance by some practitioners, it's also a practice of purifying your body and soul (according to the religious approach).

11. Better Mental Performance

Intermittent fasting enhances the cognitive function and also is very useful when it comes to boosting your brainpower. There are several factors of intermittent fasting which can support this claim. First of all, it increases the level of brain-derived neurotrophic factor (also known as BDNF), a protein in your brain that can interact with the parts of your brain responsible for controlling cognitive and memory functions, as well as learning. BDNF can even protect and stimulate the growth of new brain cells. Through IF, you will enter the ketosis state, during which your body turns fat into energy, by using ketones. Ketones can also feed your brain, and therefore improve your mental acuity, productivity, and energy.

12. Activating Cellular Repair

Fasting has been known to kick-start the body's natural cellular repair function, get rid of mature cells, increase longevity, and improve hormone function. All things that tend to become problems as people age. This can alleviate joint and muscle aches, as well as lower back pain. As the cells are being repaired and the damage is undone, it helps with the skin's elasticity and health.

13. Alleviates Oxidative Stress and Inflammation

Oxidative stress is when the body has an imbalance of antioxidants and free radicals. This imbalance can cause both tissue and cell damage in overweight and aging people. It can also lead to various chronic illnesses like cancer, heart disease, diabetes, and has an impact on the signs of aging. Oxidative stress can trigger the inflammation that causes these diseases.

Intermittent fasting can provide your system with a reboot that helps to alleviate oxidative stress and inflammation in middle-aged women. It also significantly reduces the risk of oxidative stress and inflammation for those overweight or obese.

14. Help to Prevent Cancer

Women over the age of 50 are at a higher risk of developing some kinds of cancers. Intermittent fasting, as shown in research, can cut off some of the pathways that lead to cancer. It can also help slow down the rate at which an existing tumor grows in the body.

15. Helps with Sleep and Clarity

Hormonal changes in the body can cause one's sleeping pattern to be destabilized, especially around the post-menstrual age. Many older women have testified how the intermittent fasting lifestyle has improved their sleeping patterns. If you're currently experiencing sleep issues, intermittent fasting is an option for you.

16. Boosts Productivity

Growing old can be quite a tedious stage of life for people struggling with their health daily. It could rob them of the joy of living, experiencing life, and getting things done. Older people are happier when they can stay fit and healthy. Retirement doesn't mean you are bored! There are many things you might want to do with your life at that point, and activities that could bring you fulfillment if you're healthy enough to partake in them.

CHAPTER 3

THE PROBLEM OF
EATING IN MENOPAUSE

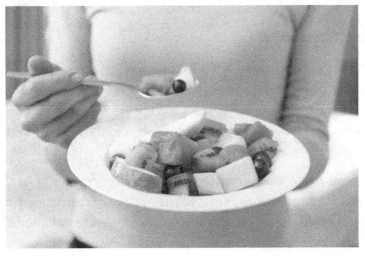

Menopause is one of the most complicated phases in a woman's life. It is the time when our bodies begin to change and important natural transitions occur that are too often negatively affected, so it is important to learn how to change our eating habits and eating patterns appropriately. In fact, it often happens that a woman is not ready for this new condition and experiences it with a feeling of defeat as an inevitable sign of time travel, and this feeling of prostration turns out to be too invasive and involves many aspects of one's stomach.

Therefore, it is important to remain calm as soon as there are messages about the first signs of change in our body, to ward off the onset of menopause for the right purpose and to minimize the negative effects of suffering, especially in the early days. Even during this difficult transition, targeted nutrition can be very beneficial.

17. What Happens to the Body of a Menopausal Woman?

It must be said that a balanced diet has been carried out in life and there are no major weight fluctuations, this will undoubtedly be a factor that supports women who are going through menopause, but that it is not a sufficient condition to present with classic symptoms that are felt, which can be classified according to the period experienced. In fact, we can distinguish between the pre-menopausal phase, which is around 45 to 50 years and is physiologically compatible with a drastic reduction in the production of estrogen hormone (responsible for the menstrual cycle, which actually starts irregularly). This period is accompanied by a series of complex and highly subjective endocrine changes. Compare effectively: headache, depression, anxiety, and sleep disorders.

When someone enters actual menopause, estrogen hormone production decreases even more dramatically, the range of the symptoms widens, leading to large amounts of the hormone, for example, to a certain class called catecholamine adrenaline. The result of these changes is a dangerous heat wave, increased sweating, and the presence of tachycardia, which can be more or less severe.

However, the changes also affect the female genital organs, with the volume of the breasts, uterus, and ovaries decreasing. The mucous membranes become less active and vaginal dryness increases. There may also be changes in bone balance, with decreased calcium intake and increased mobilization at the expense of the skeletal system. Because of this, there is a lack of continuous bone formation, and conversely, erosion begins, which is a predisposition for osteoporosis.

Although menopause causes major changes that greatly change a woman's body and soul, metabolism is one of the worst. In fact, during menopause, the absorption and accumulation of sugars and triglycerides changes and it is easy to increase some clinical values such as cholesterol and triglycerides, which lead to high blood pressure or arteriosclerosis. In addition, many women often complain of disturbing circulatory disorders and local edema, especially in the stomach. It also makes weight gain easier, even though you haven't changed your eating habits.

18. The Ideal Diet for Menopause

In cases where disorders related to the arrival of menopause become difficult to manage, drug or natural therapy under medical supervision may be necessary. The contribution given by a correct diet at this time can be considerable, in fact, given the profound variables that come into play, it is necessary to modify our food routine, both in order not to be surprised by all these changes, and to adapt in the most natural way possible.

The problem of fat accumulation in the abdominal area is always caused by the drop in estrogen. In fact, they are also responsible for the classic hourglass shape of most women, which consists of depositing fat mainly on the hips, which begins to fail with menopause. As a result, we go from a gynoid condition to an android one, with an adipose increase localized on the belly. In addition, the metabolic rate of disposal is reduced, this means that even if you do not change your diet and eat the same quantities of food as you always do, you could experience weight gain, which will be more marked in the presence of bad habits or irregular diet.

The digestion is also slower and intestinal function becomes more complicated. This further contributes to swelling, as well as the occurrence of intolerance and digestive disorders that have never been disturbed before. Therefore, the beginning will be more problematic and difficult to manage during this period. The distribution of nutrients must be different: reducing the amount of low carbohydrate, which is always preferred not to be purified, helps avoid the peak of insulin and at the same time maintains stable blood sugar.

Furthermore, it will be necessary to slightly increase the quantity of both animal and vegetable proteins; choose good fats, preferring seeds and extra-virgin olive oil, and severely limit saturated fatty acids (those of animal origin such as lard, etc.). All this to try to increase the proportion of antioxidants taken, which will help to counteract the effect of free radicals, whose concentration begins to increase during this period. It will be necessary to prefer foods rich in phytoestrogens, which will help to control the states of stress to which the body is subjected and which will favor, at least in part, the overall estrogenic balance.

These molecules are divided into three main groups and the foods that contain them should never be missing on our tables: isoflavones, present mainly in legumes such as soy and red clover; lignans, of which flax seeds and oily seeds, in general, are particularly rich; coumestans, found in sunflower seeds, beans, and sprouts. The calcium supplementation will be necessary through cheeses such as Parmesan; dairy products such as yogurt, egg yolk, some vegetables such as rocket, Brussels sprouts, broccoli, spinach, asparagus; legumes; dried fruit such as nuts, almonds, or dried grapes.

Excellent additional habits that will help to regain well-being may be: limiting sweets to sporadic occasions, thus drastically reducing sugars (for example by giving up sugar in coffee and getting used to drinking it bitterly); learn how to dose alcohol a lot (avoiding spirits, liqueurs, and aperitif drinks) and choose only one glass of good wine when you are in company, this because it tends to increase visceral fat, which is precisely what is going to settle at the abdominal level. Clearly, even by eating lots of fruit, it is difficult to reach a high carbohydrate quota as in a traditional diet. However, a dietary plan to follow can be useful to have a more precise indication on how to distribute the foods. Obviously, one's diet must be structured in a personal way, based on specific metabolic needs and one's lifestyle.

19. Perimenopause

There are many ways to lose weight during perimenopause, such as intuitive eating, a low-carb diet, a ketogenic diet, and more. If you are experiencing menopausal symptoms along with an unhealthy lifestyle (i.e., high intake of carbs, sugar, or processed foods), then you may need help in other areas as well (exercising regularly) before choosing an approach. Trying several different approaches may lead you to the ideal approach for your body and life stage.

Understanding your perimenopausal symptoms will help you determine which dietary approach and exercise regimen is best for you. If you find any of the following signs, then these should be your first concern:

- Aging or weight gain
- Significant mood swings or depression
- Low libido, hot flashes, night sweats, or difficulty sleeping
- Difficulty concentrating, memory loss, impatience, and irritability
- Constantly tired or needing caffeine after lunch to wake up in the afternoon

These are not all the signs associated with perimenopause—there are many others.

20. Intermittent Fasting Benefits—Introduction to Perimenopause

The three main strategies you have for managing perimenopausal symptoms include diet, exercise, and supplements. There are many different eating habits that may contribute to weight loss during this time. Some of these include paleo, vegetarian, and vegan diets (low-fat). If you already follow a certain diet plan (such as a low-carb or ketogenic diet), then a modified version of it may be more effective. For example, if you follow a whole food plant-based diet (WFPB), then try eating WFPB more—but less—than usual on fast days. This may provide you with the most significant benefits. If this is the case, then you can eat whole plant foods as normal on non-fast days. In this way, your body and hormones will not be shocked by a sudden change in your diet or lifestyle.

More information on perimenopause and healthy options can be found on our website. Our nutritionists are happy to answer your questions and help you determine the best path for you.

CHAPTER 4

HOW DOES INTERMITTENT FASTING WORK?

Before we can fully grasp how intermittent fasting works, we must know that there are only two states in which the body can be. They are; the fed and fasted state.

In other words, the body is in the state of reserving food energy or of utilizing or expending reserved energy. The primary goal of intermittent fasting is to ensure there is a balance in these two states.

Here is what happens during the fed state. When we consume food, the food goes through metabolism and then produces energy. Some of this energy is immediately spent, while some are reserved.

The reservation of energy is a vital responsibility of a hormone called insulin. So, during the fed state (that is, the eating period), insulin increases to break down carbohydrates first into simple sugar units known as glucose. This glucose is what the body immediately converts into its fuel, which is known as adenosine triphosphate (ATP)—this process is known as catabolism.

Secondly, in other to store more energy, it then builds up glucose in glycogen, which is a more complex form of sugar. This process is known as anabolism. This built-up energy is stored in the liver and sometimes muscles get broken down later into glucose (the form of energy the body can easily use).

However, the body doesn't have an unlimited storage capacity to continue storing glycogen. So, what happens when it hits its trench hold? The body initiates a process known as de novo lipogenesis. This process is used to store more glucose by simply converting excess glucose into fat.

In this form, the body has an unlimited storage capacity. Some of this newly converted fat could be stored in the liver, but a bulk of the fat is moved and stored all over the body. This is known as body fat, and it results in weight gain.

On the other hand, during the fasted state (that is, the period without eating), the body carries out the opposite process. The body reduces the production of insulin, which we know is responsible for the storage of energy. Once the insulin level drops, the body immediately knows its state has changed and therefore its process must change.

The body, knowing very well that there is no food coming in and hence no external source of energy, is forced to visit its reserve. The body at this state begins to carry out catabolism. First, it starts breaking down glucose that was formerly stored in complex forms as glycogen.

The energy released in that process can sustain the body for up to 36 hours. If the body continues in this state, it is further forced to start breaking down its fat reserve. This mode that the body enters is called ketosis. It is the stage where the body switches from its usual and normal source of energy, which is glucose, to ketones and fat.

With this, the body can have the energy to function for days depending on the amount of already accumulated fat. This process would result in weight loss naturally.

When one intermittently fasts, they are only creating or maintaining the balance between the fed state and the fasted state. An imbalance may be in the side of always eating, which causes the body to have more calories than it really needs. Aside from that, it also continuously overworks the body as it continuously breaks down consumed food.

This could result in several health issues. So, in order to remain healthy, one must, from time to time, frequently allow the body to use up its reserved fat. This is absolutely normal as all animals do it to maintain their health.

21. How Intermittent Fasting Affects the Brain

The brain is a vital organ responsible for controlling every other part of the body. And it will interest you to know that the human brain makes up less than 2% of the total body mass. It is the principal seat of intelligence and is responsible for our personal and societal developments.

Among the numerous functions of the brain include; maintaining consciousness, memory recall, process data including languages, skill learning, and so on. So, the importance of ensuring that the necessary nutrients needed by the brain are provided cannot be overemphasized.

To keep the brain healthy and functioning at an optimal level, the brain uses up to about 20% of the calories generated each day. For such a small organ as the brain, one would think this amount of energy is too much. But the brain is always working, sending signals throughout the body.

The signals sent by the brain either bring about voluntary actions or involuntary actions. Even when we are asleep, the brain still works, although not as much as when we are fully awake.

If the brain needs this much energy to function, the next thing that might come to mind is that fasting would have a negative effect on it. But this is not true, as we will begin to examine how fasting works when it has to do with the brain. First of all, fasting plays an important role in the development of new brain cells.

When we intermittently fast, the brain-derived neurotrophic factor (BDNF) is triggered, which facilitates the process of developing synapses and brain cells. Fasting also enhances serotonin, which is a chemical messenger in the brain. BDNF is commonly known to prevent stroke and depression.

Fasting increases these functions and a lot more of BDNF up to about 55 to 350%. Another way fasting affects the brain is that it works to prevent neurodegeneration. We already know that fasting initiates autophagy, and during this process, beta-amyloid plaques are evacuated from the body, thus reducing oxidative stress, which might be on the neuronal tissue. Fasting has been reported to be one of the treatments for epileptic patients.

Intermittent fasting not only prevents degeneration but also enhances neuroregeneration and protection. This is done by boosting growth hormones, which act to prevent muscle depreciation. Lastly, fasting helps to facilitate mitochondrial biogenesis, which is known as the powerhouse of the cell.

The brain contains numerous cells and, as such, contains numerous mitochondria. A boost in mitochondria results in an increase of available energy in the brain. However, this will be discussed in detail below. Still, there is a wide range of beliefs that fasting causes starvation, which in turn leads to hypoglycemia.

This is the survival state of the body—instead of the body starting to convert saved glucose and subsequently stored fat in the body, the body continues to store up this energy and enters into a hibernation mode. At this stage, the blood sugar drops, and the body starts to shut down some of its functions.

The individual starts experiencing fatigue, shivers, low brain function in the form of forgetfulness, and lastly, fainting. While this might be true for extended unmonitored fasting, this is not the case for intermittent fasting. The reason is that, eventually, one eats after avoiding food for some time. So, the body knows it has not gotten to starvation.

22. How Intermittent Fasting Affects the Mitochondria

Like we noted earlier, mitochondria are the powerhouse of the cells. Their health is very important not only for the cell but for the entire organism. To ensure the mitochondria (and the entire cell) remain in good health, dysfunctional cellular components that eventually cause inflammation must be eliminated.

Also, the cell needs to perpetually be in homeostasis, and free radicals, either chemicals or organelles, cannot be allowed to remain in the cell. All these processes can be triggered by time-controlled fasting.

Intermittent fasting can also engineer the development of new mitochondria through the process of mitochondria biogenesis. This process is a result of some metabolic regulators, which include AMPK and PGC-1.

The regulators are responsible for not only building new mitochondria but also regulating mitophagy (the process where the mitochondria self-heals). They initiate the building of new mitochondria by sending signals to the body to increase the production of more energy in a stressful and energy-depleting environment (intermittent fasting).

To follow this command, the cell then develops new mitochondria (power plants) to produce more energy. This process has the effect of keeping one always energized and youthful.

It also boosts mitochondria density. This is the ability of the mitochondria to not just produce more energy while making use of fewer resources but to be very efficient in doing it. This development is a result of a boost in NAD+ levels, which is one function of intermittent fasting.

The NAD+ is an enzyme that plays a vital role for the mitochondria to be able to produce more energy. Its presence in the cell energizes the mitochondria in its early stages of life. It also restores and replenishes the mitochondria during old age. This is done by initiating mitophagy as well as DNA repair.

Another key function of the NAD+ is the activation of Sirtuins. Sirtuins are charged with the responsibility of protecting the cell from stress. Like we mentioned earlier, during an IF, the body begins to burn stored body fat instead of its regular glucose.

The breaking down of glucose leaves behind free radicals and produces higher oxidative stress when compared to breaking down fatty acids. So, we can say that intermittent fasting slows down mitochondria's aging process because it leads to the release of way fewer free radicals and oxidative stress in the cell.

23. How Intermittent Fasting Affects the Immune System

The immune system is essential in the body as its health ensures the whole body's continued health. When fasting, stem cells are turned on. These stem cells play vital roles in rejuvenating aging cells, which end up prolonging their youthfulness. An example of this stem cell is the Hematopoietic Stem Cell (HSC).

Fasting accomplishes this process by shutting down Cyclic Adenosine Monophosphate (cAMP), dependent Protein Kinase A (PKA). The cAMP is a molecule messenger, while PKA is a bunch of enzymes. Both are responsible for the regulation of fat, glycogen, and sugar metabolism.

Once PKA is shut down by turning on the cAMP signal, the body knows to start mobilizing its reserved energy. And the minute the body begins to burn body fat, stem cells are activated. But it takes time for this process to start.

This is because the body needs to finish burning all available glucose and all the glycogen it reserved before it can then begin to burn body fat reserve. So, for this to happen, one has to engage in regular or long-term intermittent fasting.

Also, fasting could act as stressors that could be harmful to the body. But if it is done correctly in time, it can become a handy tool. Gradually exposing the body to stressors through intermittent fasting helps the body get used to and develop resilience against them.

So, the more one intermittently fasts, the more resilient to stressors one's immune system becomes.

CHAPTER 5

HISTORY OF
INTERMITTENT FASTING

Often confused with starvation, fasting is not a recent concept; it is as old as the known human history. It is completely natural and much needed for body development. Even the word "breakfast" itself indicates that we normally fast between two meals of the day. Intermittent fasting takes this process to the next step and sets up a dietary routine that works best for the body's health.

Fasting, in one form or another, remained widely prevalent in every ancient civilization because of its obvious benefits. We often hear stories of monks acquiring spiritual superiority and physical strength through fasts. The tradition existed even during 460 to 370 BC, the times of Hippocrates, who is considered today the pioneer of modern medicine. He prescribed two basic methods to achieve physical healing: one was fasting and the other was the intake of apple cider vinegar.

"To eat when you are sick is to feed your illness"—(Hippocrates of Kos)

Those words of Hippocrates laid the basis of intermittent fasting, which is equally relevant today. His ideas about fasting and its benefits were also shared by other Greek physicians and writers of the time like Plutarch, who, between 46–120 AD, preached the concept of fasting by describing it as a better approach to treat illness than the use of medicines. Likewise, other great names of Greece, Aristotle and Plato, also supported the concept of fasting and implemented it during their lifetimes.

According to the ancient Greek experts, fasting can be described as the 'physician within' oneself because when a person falls ill, the body naturally loses the appetite to eat, which means that healing can be carried out when a person is fasting. Feeling anorexic when you are sick is natural, and only supports the need for fasting. Thus, with the historical evidence alongside a biological understanding of the human body, it can be inferred that fasting is an essential requirement of every individual and helps in improving health. Besides physical fitness, fasting was also considered an effective means of boosting the cognitive potential of a person, according to Greek physicists. When a person is on the fast, the body and mind go into an ultra-alter mode as most of the blood is supplied to the brain instead of the digestive system. This is the reason why a person feels drowsy and lethargic when he consumes a large amount of food at a time because all the energy and the blood are supplied to digest the food.

Another great supporter of fasting is the founder of toxicology, Philip Paracelsus, who followed in the footsteps of Hippocrates and Galen by writing excessively about the benefits of fasting. He also termed it the internal physician, the greatest remedy. Moving forward to the modern medicinal history of America, from 1706–1790, Benjamin Franklin also highlighted fasting and resting as two better approaches than medicine.

Fasting is also supported by almost all the major religions in the world. Therefore, we find that the respective followers in each religious cult are keeping fasts. According to different religions like Christianity, Jainism, Hinduism, Buddhism, and Islam, fasting is directly linked to spiritual upliftment. It is also described as a means of getting control of the body and its desires. This is where religion and science meet when it comes to fasting, a better control of the body means a person can make wise and healthy food choices for oneself.

Though fasting has always been in use, the contemporary approach of intermittent fasting emerged in 2012, when it was readily picked up by health experts all around the world, and is now widely recommended to people suffering from different health issues. It all started with one single documentary "Eat Fast, Live longer and Book the Fast diet," presented by Dr. Michael Mosley. He was followed by Kate Harrison who wrote a complete book on one of the fasting methods, named the 5:2 diet. Soon in 2016, Dr. Jason Fung stepped up with his book "The Obesity Code," which was also marked as the bestseller of that year. In his book, Fung extensively wrote about his own experience with intermittent fasting and how it can be most effective by pairing it with a suitable healthy diet. He recommended the use of fresh vegetables, fruits, protein-rich food, low-carb items, and intake of healthy fats in the diet.

Steadily, all this work on intermittent fasting made enough buzz that people, in general, started opting for its various approaches. Initially, it was just television or movie celebrities who followed the fasting patterns. Then they became the source of inspiration for millions of people.

CHAPTER 6

---❖---

WHAT IS A MEAL PLAN?

A meal plan is a means to keep your eating on track with your goals. There are a few variables to keep in mind. How much time do you have to prepare the meals? What keeps best in the refrigerator at work, if you work? How much can you make ahead of time, say Sunday afternoon, which will last the entire week?

24. The essential Intermittent Fasting Meal Plan for Beginners

If you are new to fasting, starting by just eating for a long time, from 8 a.m. to 6 p.m., is an excellent method to dunk your toes into the fasting waters. This arrangement permits you to eat each meal in addition to specific snacks, and at the same time, get in 14 hours of fasting inside a 24-hour term.

Breakfast: at 8 a.m., drink a Green Smoothie.

After fasting, start drinking a smoothie, since it is somewhat more straightforward for the gut to process. You'll need to go for a green smoothie rather than a high-sugar natural product smoothie to abstain from beginning your day on an exciting glucose ride. Include heaps of solid fats to prop you up until lunch!

Lunch: at midnight, eat Grass-Fed Burgers.

Grass-fed liver burgers are preferred for lunch during the week, and they are straightforward to prepare. The burgers are served on a layer of dark leafy greens with a dressing for supper pressed with B nutrients for solid methylation and detox pathways.

Dinner: at 5:30 p.m., eat Salmon and Veggies.

Salmon is an excellent source of omega-3 fats. Green veggies like kale and broccoli have high anti-oxidative properties.

Other alternatives, respect salmon, can be any wild-caught fish based on your personal preference. Serve a portion of your preferred vegetables cooked in coconut oil, and you have a simple superfood.

CHAPTER 7

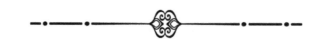

HOW TO SET UP A SUCCESS MEAL PLAN
IN INTERMITTENT FASTING

25. Foods to Eat for Women over 50 in Intermittent Fasting

The dietary needs of a fifty-year-old woman are very different from those of younger females. Your body requires slightly different foods and nutrition than those of teenage females and even middle-aged women. Therefore, you will need to know what works and what doesn't.

The reason why I am dedicating an entire part of foods to eat is because the need arises. You need to know what food you will be eating and how it is going to benefit you. Furthermore, you will know that despite having a long list of foods to avoid, there are still a number of food items that you can enjoy at this age. Just because you have turned fifty or near doesn't mean you don't get to enjoy your life. With proper care, life will still be good with much to offer.

The physiological impacts that are present in your age have long-term health effects. Quite possibly you may not be taking care of those critical things right now since they are not seemingly important. However, little things add up and in your case, they will have long-term effects. Therefore, you need to pack your gear and start a journey of self-care. With little effort in your daily habits, you will end up being a healthy fifty-year-old woman with the grace of a thirty-year-old or even younger.

Before you read this, I would ask that you consult a health professional or dietician regarding your needs. Quite possibly you may not be allowed to certain meats or fruits and here it might be mentioned. The entire list of foods that I have given is for general women above fifty. Make sure you aren't allergic to one of the foods given below or it is not harmful to you.

26. What Kind of Food Requirements Should You Have?

At this age, your metabolism is not going to be as efficient as before. You will know that by the changes your body is going through. Some foods will have a reaction they never had before. Similarly, your bones are going to lose their density. Your bones will become weaker than before. It is quite interesting that there is no one diet that is going to be efficient for you. However, the healthy meal plan and the diet pattern are going to do wonders for you. Therefore, you have to make sure you achieve this.

Given below are the kinds of food types you need as a woman over the age of fifty. The foods that you should be eating will fall into one of four categories given below:

Foods that Satisfy Daily Calorie Needs

Your body processes calories slower than before. This is in direct link to the slow metabolism. Since calories are going to be burned slower than before, you are going to need fewer calories. This is because when you were younger, you would have needed more calories since your body was growing. However, at this stage, your body has reached a certain stage. It processes things slow and calories are one of them. Therefore, you don't need as much as you did when you were thirty or twenty. You need about 1800 calories to maintain your weight. Some women eat lesser than before. However, some also overeat, which is not a good habit.

The foods that satisfy your calorie requirement are the ones you should be eating. You should make sure to have nutrient-dense foods that satisfy your hunger. Some of these foods are:

- Vegetables
- Fresh Fruits
- Lean Meats
- Fish
- Beans and Legumes
- Nuts and seeds
- Eggs
- Dairy

While some of the most common snack items may include potato and chips, as well as processed foods, I wouldn't recommend eating them too much. Sweetened beverages, crackers, or foods containing a high amount of sodium or fats needed to be kept in check.

Foods that Support Hormone Changes

I will not lie. Menopause is hell and the hormone changes that you experience can easily throw you off balance. There are many side effects such as night sweats, hot flashes, unpredictable mood swings, and much more. These are usually the symptoms of pre-menopause and post-menopause. While females don't want to try intermittent fasting during menopause, you need to make sure you get these foods. Females try to lose weight. When you do intermittent fasting after menopause, make sure to get these foods properly.

The first ingredient that promises good hormone changes is omega-3 fatty acid. These particular nutrients can be found in cold-water fish like salmon, sardines, and tuna. Among the foods that provide their natural supply, flax seeds are also included. The flax seeds also supply a type of fiber that is helpful during hot flashes. Furthermore, as the list extends, you will also need to consider soy foods.

The soy foods such as soymilk, tofu, and similar other food items are also very helpful. The menopausal symptoms are eased by eating soy foods.

Foods for Bone Health

As females have turned fifty, the bones become less dense and they start lacking in nutrients. This makes the bones weaker than before. As such, a diet containing vitamin D and calcium is generally preferred. As a woman over the age of fifty, you will find that yogurt, cow's milk, goat's milk, cheese, and similar foods are generally a big yes for you. There are also many vegetables that are rich in calcium. You will end up needing all of them. Generally, your main goal is getting Vitamin D and the sunlight is going to provide you that. In fact, getting more sunlight is the best way to get vitamin D naturally. You may also take vitamin D supplements. However, make sure before you start anything, you consult your doctor.

Antioxidants Foods

You need foods that will help you ward off free radicals. These are rogue molecules that are formed as you age towards your fifties. The free radicals' molecules damage cells and decrease your immunity. The immunity if decreased will make you more vulnerable against the diseases. Consequently, you should be eating foods that have a high content of Vitamin C. Mostly the citrus fruits are one of those types.

27. List of General Foods That Satisfy the Calorie Needs

I have thoroughly researched the list of foods that you are supposed to consume. With aging, our diet needs to be healthy and well balanced. There is no one food that is a general one, satisfying all of your requirements. Furthermore, there is no one-size-fits-all food. Certain foods and diets will be repeated, making you aware of their multiple uses. Furthermore, you should know that as a woman over the age of fifty, your entire focus needs to be on your health. Let us first look at the list of foods.

The first big change that you will need to make is to eat more fruits and vegetables. Some of those fruits will be well explained in the list I am about to give you. Some people suggest that eating canned food is the same as eating raw vegetables or fruits. I would disagree. As a woman over the age of fifty, I would recommend you purchase fresh stock from a farmer's market or nearby shop. You should turn your focus more on eating leafy green vegetables. Most leafy green vegetables include lettuce, cabbage, and similar vegetables. You can also eat dark green vegetables and reap their full benefit. An example of a dark green vegetable is broccoli. Among colored vegetables, I would highly recommend orange vegetables such as carrots or sweet potatoes.

I already explained how your body needs more proteins. As a woman over the age of fifty, you automatically fall into the category of elder people. For you, needing protein means needing more meat and fish. However, some women misunderstand that the protein is only present in fish. You should eat a balanced diet of beans and peas too since they also contain proteins. Vary your diet between fish and beans along with peas.

This is the perfect time to start measuring your diet. You should eat at least three ounces of whole-grain cereals, pasta, bread or rice. Crackers can also fit into this category as long as they have been made healthily. You should eat these three ounces every day. Make sure it is present either in your breakfast, lunch, or dinner. You can also break it down and include it in both meals of intermittent fasting.

Fat-free dairy is a must! Have three servings of them in your diet. I would recommend milk as I will mention in some of the foods I will give below. Replace the dense-fat dairy with low-fat dairy. You can also use olive oil or coconut oil where possible in your diet.

You should switch from solid fats to light fats. Make sure to utilize low-fat cooking oil.

Make sure to get plenty of vitamin B-12. It can be easily found in lean meats, eggs, and milk. This particular vitamin is used for enhancing your brain functions that is normally a requirement of elder people, including ladies over the age of fifty. Make sure to take a limited supply of eggs or meats that have high cholesterol content in them.

28. Diet Plan for Women Over 50

As you will have noticed, there are many fasting techniques. However, it is not always easy to choose which one is right for us. In addition, it is sometimes difficult to know what to eat during the intermittent fasting period.

Lunch / Dinner Menu

Intermittent fasting does not prevent hydration. Therefore, it is quite possible for you to drink a large glass of water upon waking up. It is also possible to drink a cup of green tea, without sugar of course!

Lunch

A green salad as a starter. You can decorate it with raw vegetables of your choice (fennel, cucumber, radish, celery, etc.). If you want to add dressing, consider making it homemade!

White meat or white flesh fish. Accompany your meat or fish with green vegetables (green beans, peas, zucchini, etc.).

A portion of cheese or yogurt.

A fruit of your choice.

Dinner

Vegetable soup. It is obviously better to prepare your soup yourself. If you are not the soup pro, don't panic!

White meat or white flesh fish. Accompany your meat or fish with a small portion of starchy foods (pasta, rice, etc.).

A white cheese.

A fruit of your choice.

Dinner / Breakfast Menu

Breakfast

Black coffee, green tea or herbal tea without sugar.

A bowl of cereal or porridge.

Some almonds with a choice of yogurt.

Dinner

Vegetable soup. You can prepare your soup yourself, it is better. Don't worry if you are not a pro!

White meat or white flesh fish. You can accompany them with a small portion of starchy foods (pasta, rice, etc.) or green vegetables (green beans, peas, zucchini, etc.).

A portion of cheese.

A fruit of your choice.

CHAPTER 8

HOW TO INCREASE YOUR ENERGY
THANKS TO INTERMITTENT FASTING

Hormones can equally affect a person's energy levels. During menstrual cycles, energy levels have been known to spike and rise due to increased levels of estrogen. After the menstrual cycle, the levels of estrogen drop quite drastically causing lethargy. As women reach menopause and estrogen levels start to drop, women feel less energetic and extremely tired.

Another hormonal culprit that contributes to a menopausal woman's lack of energy is progesterone. This hormone declines with age and is one of the reasons middle-aged women have problems sleeping. Progesterone is used to induce ovulation in younger women, but it also promotes sleep. Obviously, a woman going through middle age no longer has the need of ovulation, so her body does not produce as much as it used to.

Although they do not produce it in the amounts a man does, a woman's body also produces testosterone. Testosterone performs a significant role in the production of red blood cells in the body. Red blood cells are the cells that transport oxygen around the body, which is a much-needed component in the promotion of energy. As with many other hormones, menopause limits the production of testosterone as well.

High stress levels will cause an increase in cortisol, you will that it know keeps a person awake. This affects sleep patterns, which is just another added factor causing a lack of energy due to feeling tired. It will also have an impact on a woman's mood and leave them feeling horrible.

There are ways to increase energy levels, but the first step to take is to measure your hormone levels. This can be done by your medical advisor, a registered clinic, or there are home tests you can buy at the drugstore. Ask a pharmacist what the best and most reliable brands are. Once you know what you are dealing with, there are a few methods you can try to increase energy levels.

Never try hormone replacements or balancing hormones without the advice of a medical professional. If you are not on any medication or have any pre-existing medical conditions, you can try one of the following tips:

- Ask your doctor, nutritionist, or pharmacist to recommend a good quality multi-vitamin. Make sure you fall into a routine of taking them.

- Slowly change your diet to one that offers more nutrition and agrees with your system. As you age, you will find foods that you may no longer be able to eat.

- Find a quiet time to take ten to fifteen minutes to meditate, clear your mind, and learn the art of breathing. Tibetan monks have practiced Anapanasati, which is mindfulness through breathing.

- Get enough good-quality sleep. You may need to make some adjustments to your bedroom. Make sure your pillow is supporting your head and that your mattress is doing the same for your body. Take all electronics out of your room; if you use your mobile phone for an alarm, make sure it goes into sleep mode. Instead of a TV, make room for a chair to curl up in and read. Reading before bed is a great way to unwind and slip into another world to clear your mind. Try not to take naps during the day.

- Get in some exercise at least once a day, twice if you can manage it. It does not mean you have to go running a marathon or do the "Tour de France." Go for a walk, do some gardening, or take a gentle bike ride and look at the scenery.

- Find a new hobby or take up an old one you had put aside. If you engage your mind, you will automatically gear your body up for action.

- There are supplements and certain foods to naturally boost your energy. Whatever you do, do not try highly caffeinated drinks, or other such types of energy boosters you find in a supermarket.

By now, you will know the next bit of advice is going to be: drink lots of water. It is a great cure for a whole lot of things including lethargy. If you want to get a little extra boost, try using an icepack on your Vagus nerve in your neck for a minute at a time.

CHAPTER 9

EXERCISE AND GYM WORKOUT TO MATCH WITH THE INTERMITTENT FASTING DIET

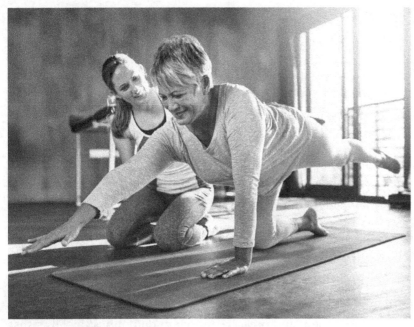

As with all forms of weight loss diets, intermittent fasting can only maximize its results if paired with some form of physical exercise. The situation is slightly different when we are talking about individuals over the age of fifty, as the first priority, in this case, will be the overall health of the person.

What most people fear is the potential of hurting their joints and ligaments, which tend to become more sensible with age. Indeed, this is an underlying factor that cannot be neglected, but it does not exclude all forms of exercise.

When we hear about physical training, the first thought rushed towards the image of a gym, intense workouts, and exhaustion. However, people over the age of fifty do not stop working. You might have a physically demanding job, a lifestyle that includes long walks, or even a passion for activities such as yoga.

Although lower on intensity, these are all forms of exercise that ultimately move you towards the general goal, burning calories. We do not need to overdo the concept of exercise beyond the point where it gets destructive for our joints, unlike the popular belief that we have to push our bodies to their limits.

There are certain activities that can act as exercise and aid in both the weight loss effects of intermittent fasting and also bring a whole new variety of benefits, such as, but not limited to, preserving joint and ligament health.

Some of these include yoga, as it is not only a light form of exercise, but women, in particular, enjoy the activity on a general basis. You do not need to go to specialized classes in order to engage in this activity, as the internet bears plenty of material regarding art.

The reason we urge you to give yoga classes a try is the sensation of a group activity, which motivates many and brings more enjoyment to the table. Our main focus is continuity, and if you can find a yoga class where you end up feeling great in the community, this whole process will become even more enjoyable.

Not only that, but most classes have participants with a shared interest, and it should come as no surprise if you happen to stumble upon other women who engage in intermittent fasting, giving you space to share your knowledge in return for more knowledge. The supportive nature of organized classes, as well as their popularity nowadays and the sensation of community, make this a great option if you are interested in taking your results to the next level, and perhaps discovering a new hobby.

If you find yoga somehow unfitting for your personal needs, we need to point out another activity that acts in great effect to protect your ligaments, which is swimming.

Swimming is a wonderful sport as it can be done at varying levels of intensity, according to the person, and aids with preserving joint health and mobility. The question is easy in terms of opportunity, do you enjoy swimming?

If the answer is yes, or you used to enjoy it, going for a few laps once or twice a week will work wonders in terms of boosting your health. It is not overly exhausting, yet provides sufficient stimulus to preserve musculature and keep it safe from the effects of aging in the long term.

Combined with the number of calories it burns, as well as the cardiovascular effects, this form of mild exercise will be the cornerstone of your health, as it also helps to prevent cardiovascular disease, blood pressure problems, and a variety of muscle, bone, and joint issues.

Last but not least, certain gyms feature special classes for people with more advanced age, which focus on light to mild exercises, meant to help you lose weight and preserve muscle and joint health. All of that under the supervision and guidance of a specialized trainer, to make sure all of the workouts are conducted safely.

If neither yoga nor swimming seem attractive to you, this is the last more unique form of physical exercise we have to recommend. Just like with yoga classes, the sensation provided by group workouts and the presence of people similar to you and with share interests can make this environment highly constructive.

As a last mention, if you are uninterested in doing any of the activities listed above, the only small tweak we still have to remind you of is a lot more convenient and milder, yet still effective.

Opting to walk instead of commuting by car or bus whenever possible can make quite a difference, as it burns added calories, mobilizes the legs, and is generally an enjoyable activity.

The fact is, any form of added physical work is going to act in the way you want it to, and as the primary objective is healthy weight loss, we need to focus extensively on the health part.

These activities are amazing for doing just that, and are optimal in order to develop new hobbies, making the weight loss and health-boosting process so much more enjoyable. With that, we are closing this section of the book, with one last idea to mention.

Regular gym workouts under a personal trainer should not be excluded, as most trainers are experienced in working with women over the age of forty or fifty, more than you'd imagine. The downside comes in the cost and intensity these training routines have and are only suitable for people who can preserve the continuity during extended periods of time.

CHAPTER 10

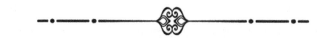

MOST COMMON MISTAKES AND ISSUES ON DOING THE INTERMITTENT FASTING DIET

The results of intermittent fasting vary from one person to the other, but overall, every individual should be able to reap some benefits from fasting. The key is doing it right, and doing it consistently. Here are some common mistakes that could compromise your outcomes:

29. Starting with an Extreme Plan

Now that you have found a fasting plan that sounds just perfect for your needs, don't you just want to jump in there with all your enthusiasm and, well, kick the hell out of it? You must be already imagining your new look after shedding those extra pounds. Can the fasting start now? Well, not so fast. Don't let your zest lead you to an intense plan that will subject your body to a drastic change. You can't come from 3 meals a day and snacks in between to a 24-hour fast. That will only leave you feeling miserable. Start with skipping single meals. Or avoiding snacks. Once your body gets used to short fasts, you can proceed to as far as your body can take, within reasonable limits. Go slow on exercising as well during the fasting phase, at least in the initial weeks, as it could cause adrenal fatigue.

30. Quitting Too Soon

Have you been fasting for a paltry one week and have already decided that it is too hard? Are you struggling with hunger pangs, cravings, mood swings, low energy levels and so on? Well, such a reaction should be anticipated. The first couple of weeks can be harsh as the body adjusts to the reduced calorie intake. You will be hungry, irritable, and exhausted. Still, you will be required to remain consistent. Even if you cannot feel it, the body is adapting to the changes. If you give up during this period and revert to normal eating, you'll just roll back on the adjustments that the body had already made. Any change requires discipline, and this one is no exception. Hang in there; things will get better with time.

31. 'Feasting' Too Much

Some quarters refer to intermittent fasting as alternating phases of fasting and feasting. This largely suggests that as soon as the clock hits the last minute of fast time, you dig right into a large savory meal, the kind that you end with a loud satisfied belch. Ideally, there should be nothing wrong with this approach, after all, you've successfully made it through your fasting window.

But remember that your main goal here is to burn fat and lose weight. That only works if you have fewer calories going in compared to those going out. The larger your meal, the higher the number of calories that you're introducing into the body.

You don't need to eat a mountain. Start with fruits and vegetables. They contain fiber that will leave you feeling fuller, so you won't need that large meal. Eat slowly, listening to the signals of getting full. Stop eating as soon as you feel full, even if there's still food on your plate, which you may have piled up due to the hunger you were feeling. Refrigerate the extra for another meal. You don't have to eat all through the eating window either. Once you're satisfied, go on and concentrate on other things.

32. Insufficient Calories

While some will overeat to make up for the 'lost time,' others will eat very little, fearing to turn back the gains already made. This results in inadequate calories, yet these calories are required to fuel the body to perform its functions optimally. With insufficient nutrients, you're likely to experience mood swings, irritability, fatigue, and low energy levels. Your day-to-day life will be compromised, and you'll be less productive. Intermittent fasting should make your life better, not worse. Eating enough will allow you to remain active, and proceed efficiently with your fasting plan.

33. Wrong Food Choices

We have already established that intermittent fasting concentrates largely on the "when" as opposed to "what" regarding eating. While that still leaves an opportunity to enjoy a wide variety of foods, it does not mean that you can eat whatever you want. Left to our own devices, most of us will go for sugary and fatty foods as they're very enticing to the taste buds. French fries, pizza, cake, cookies, candy, ice cream, processed meats, and so on. This is a very short-sighted approach though. Breaking your fast with such foods will only remove the benefits of the fast.

Go for healthy, wholesome foods that will nourish your body with all groups of nutrients. Let your meal contain adequate portions of vegetables, protein, good fats, and complex carbs. You may have heard that intermittent fasting works well with a low-carb diet. That's right, but it's a low-carb, not a no-carb diet. Some people try to accelerate weight loss by eliminating all carbs. Remember that carbs supply us with calories to fuel the body. Include a portion of healthy starch on your plate, going for brown unprocessed options where applicable.

Why should you worry about what you eat if intermittent fasting is about when you eat? Well, healthy eating is for everyone, even if you're not going through a fasting plan. You eat wholesome foods because they're good for the body, and they keep you away from lifestyle diseases. Healthy eating should be normal eating, so in this case, we can agree that the fast is accompanied by normal eating.

34. Insufficient Fluids

Staying hydrated makes your fast more tolerable. It provides you a full feeling and retains hunger pangs at bay. Fasting also breaks down the damaged components in the body, and the water helps flush them out as toxins.

You can also sip tea or coffee, with no milk or sugar added. Coffee has been known to contain compounds, which further accelerate the burning of fat. Green tea also has similar properties. You can try diverse flavors of tea or coffee to get a taste that appeals to you. As long as they don't contain any calories, they're good to go.

35. Over-Concentrating on the Eating Window

If you can't take your eyes off the clock, you're not doing it right. You can't spend the fasting phase obsessing over food, thinking of what and how much you'll eat when it's finally time. In fact, the more you think about food, the hungrier you get. That hunger you feel every 5 hours or so is emotional hunger. It is clock hunger, which you'll feel around the normal mealtimes. Real hunger mostly checks in when you've been fasting for 16 hours onwards. Get your mind off the food and concentrate on something else. If you're at home and keep circling the kitchen, leave and go somewhere else. Go to the library, for shopping (not for food of course), to the park or attend to your errands. Food is so much easier to keep away from when it's out of sight.

36. Wrong Plan

We have already been through the various fasting plans available, as well as the factors to consider when choosing a fasting plan. That should guide you to fast comfortably. How do you know that the plan you are following is not the best one for you? To begin with, the entire process becomes a major strain. You struggle with hunger, fatigue, mood swings, and low energy levels. Your performance in your duties is affected and you dread the next fast. And even after all the struggle, there's hardly any significant result to show for it. Go back and study the plans and choose one that better suits your lifestyle.

37. Stress

If you're under a great deal of stress, chances are you'll struggle through the fast. Stress causes hormone imbalances leaving you struggling with hunger pangs when you should have been fasting comfortably. Stress eating is common, characterized by cravings that drive you towards fatty and sugary foods. It also interferes with sleep, and fasting is even harder when you're not well-rested. If you've already attempted the fast and have fallen into any of these mistakes, as many often do, you can correct yourself and proceed. If you're just starting out, you now know the pitfalls to avoid. The key is to keep learning and improving, and the results will be a testament to your effort.

Managing Stress

Now that we've established that stress is one of the factors that can impair your fasting, it is imperative that you learn how to manage stress.

Here are some steps that you can take to ensure that stress does not hinder you from healthy living:

Relax Daily

Those issues that you carry in your heart and mind can cause you stress in the long run. Find a way to unwind at the end of every day so that the pressure does not build up. Watch a movie, sports, a documentary, read a book, try a new recipe, soak in the bathtub or do whatever else entertains you. Those few hours provide a positive distraction so that you can face the following day without tagging along with yesterday's challenges.

Open Up

Let somebody else know what is going on. A problem shared is half solved. Just speaking out makes you feel lighter even before you find a solution. Stress can prejudice your reasoning and judgment, making it difficult to evaluate the issues you're facing. Someone else, looking at your situation with a rational eye, will be better placed to assess the situation and suggest solutions. Speak to a family member, friend, or colleague. If you feel the matter is too personal and you prefer to speak to an expert, there are counselors available.

Get a Hobby

What is it that you enjoy doing? That thing that commands your undivided attention for hours? It could be cycling, gardening, drawing, painting, cooking, video games, and so on. Give it more time and attention. Set yourself new goals. For instance, you could challenge yourself to finish a drawing in a week, or grow a vegetable patch in a month, or knit a sweater in 3 days, or try out a new recipe every evening.

With a goal comes commitment. Now your mind will be shifted from the issues causing you to stress to something new and exciting. With every goal achieved comes a sense of accomplishment, further improving your mood. Interact with others who have a similar hobby. Join a relevant community. Even an online one will do. Take part in their activities. No matter what you're going through on any day, you have something to look forward to.

Enough Sleep

The relationship between stress and sleep is an awkward one. You're required to have enough sleep to better manage stress, yet the stress itself keeps you from sleeping. You have to look for a different trigger for sleep. Read a book, listen to music, take a relaxing shower, or whatever else soothes you to sleep. When you are well rested, you'll be better placed to evaluate the causes of your stress and possibly come up with possible solutions.

We've just spoken about making changes, right? Perhaps one of those changes that you need to make is to deactivate/suspend your account and leave the interweb for some time. Figure out your life without all the senseless pressure. Deal with people that you can show the real you and they support you. Build your life quietly and consistently. As they say, work quietly and let success make the noise.

These tips should help you control or even eliminate your stress, and you can then fast without strain.

CHAPTER 11

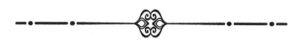

APPETIZER AND SNACK
RECIPES: 25 RECIPES

38. Low-Carb Brownies

Preparation Time: 10 minutes

Cooking Time: 20 minutes

Servings: 16

Ingredients:

- 7 tablespoons coconut oil, melted
- 6 tablespoons plant-based sweetener
- 1 large egg
- 2 egg yolk
- ½ teaspoon mint extract
- 5 ounces sugar-free dark chocolate
- ¼ cup plant-based chocolate protein powder
- 1 teaspoon baking soda
- ¼ teaspoon sea salt

- 2 tablespoons vanilla almond milk, unsweetened

Directions:

1. Start by preheating the oven to 350°F and then take an 8x8-inch pan and line it with parchment paper, being sure to leave some extra sticking up to use later to help you get them out of the pan after they are cooked.
2. Into a medium-sized vessel, use a hand mixer, and blend 5 tablespoons of the coconut oil (save the rest for later), as well as the egg, sweetener, egg yolks, and the mint extract all together for 1 minute. After this minute, the mixture will become a lighter yellow hue.

3. Take 4 ounces of the chocolate and put it in a (microwave-safe) bowl, as well as with the other 2 tablespoons of melted coconut oil.

4. Cook this chocolate and oil mixture over medium heat, at 30-second intervals, being sure to stir at each interval, just until the chocolate becomes melted and smooth.

5. While the egg mixture is being beaten, add in the melted chocolate mixture until this becomes thick and homogenous.

6. Add in your protein powder of choice, salt, baking soda, and stir until homogenous. Then, vigorously whisk your almond milk in until the batter becomes a bit smoother.

7. Finely chop the rest of your chocolate and stir these bits of chocolate into the batter you have made.

8. Spread the batter evenly into the pan you have prepared, and bake this until the edges of the batter just begin to become darker, and the center of the batter rises a little bit. You can also tell by sliding a toothpick in the middle, and when it comes out clean, it is ready. This will take approximately 20 to 21 minutes. Be sure that you do not overbake them!

9. Let them cool in the pan in which they were cooked for about 20 minutes. Then, carefully use the excess paper handles to take the brownies out of the pan and put them onto a wire cooling rack.

10. Make sure that they cool completely, and when they do, cut them, and they are ready to eat!

Nutrition:

- Calories: 107
- Fats: 10 g
- Carbohydrates: 5.7 g
- Protein: 2.5 g

39. Roasted Broccoli

Preparation Time: 5 minutes

Cooking Time: 20 minutes

Servings: 4

Ingredients:

- 4 cups broccoli florets
- 1 tablespoon olive oil
- Salt and pepper to taste

Directions:

1. Preheat your oven to 400°F.
2. Add broccoli in a zip bag alongside oil and shake until coated.
3. Add seasoning and shake again.
4. Spread broccoli out on the baking sheet, bake for 20 minutes.
5. Let it cool and serve.

Nutrition:

- Calories: 62
- **Fat:** 4 g
- Carbohydrates: 4 g
- Protein: 4 g

40. Almond Flour Muffins

Preparation Time: 15 minutes

Cooking Time: 20 minutes

Servings: 8

Ingredients:

- 1/3 cup pumpkin puree
- 3 eggs
- 2 tablespoons agave nectar
- 2 tablespoons coconut oil
- 1 teaspoon vanilla extract
- 1 teaspoon white vinegar
- 1 cup chopped fruits
- 1 teaspoon baking soda
- ½ teaspoon salt
- 2 ½ cups almond flour

Directions:

1. Preheat the oven to 350°F.
2. Line the muffin tin with paper liners
3. In the first mixing bowl, whisk the almond flour, salt, and baking soda.
4. In the second mixing bowl, whisk the pumpkin puree, eggs, coconut oil, agave nectar, vanilla extract, and vinegar.
5. Now add this puree mix of the second bowl to the first bowl and blend everything well.
6. Add the chopped fruits to the blend.
7. Pour the mixture into the muffin cups in your pan.
8. Bake for 15–20 minutes. Ensure that the contents have set in the center, and a golden-brown lining has started to appear at the edges.
9. Transfer the muffins to a cooling rack and let them cool completely.

Nutrition:

- Calories: 75
- Carbohydrates: 4 g
- **Fat:** 6 g
- Protein: 0 g

41. Squash Bites

Preparation Time: 10 minutes

Cooking Time: 40 minutes

Servings: 4

Ingredients:

- 10 ounces turkey meat, cooked, sliced
- 2 pounds butternut squash, cubed
- 1 teaspoon chili powder
- 1 teaspoon garlic powder
- 1 teaspoon sweet paprika
- Black pepper to taste

Directions:

1. In a bowl, mix butternut squash cubes with chili powder, black pepper, garlic powder, and paprika and toss to coat.
2. Wrap the squash pieces in turkey slices, place them all on a lined baking sheet, place in the oven at 350°F, bake for 20 minutes, flip and bake for 20 minutes more.
3. Arrange the squash bites on a platter and serve. Enjoy.

Nutrition:

- Calories: 223
- **Fat:** 3.8 g
- Fiber: 4.5 g
- Carbohydrates: 26.5 g
- Protein: 23 g

42. Apple Bread

Preparation Time: 10 minutes

Cooking Time: 20 minutes

Servings: 10

Ingredients:

- ½ cup honey
- ½ teaspoon nutmeg
- ½ teaspoon salt
- 1 cup applesauce, sweetened
- 1 teaspoon baking soda
- 1 teaspoon vanilla extract
- 2 ¼ cup whole wheat flour
- 2 large eggs
- 2 tablespoons vegetable oil
- 2 teaspoons baking powder
- 2 teaspoons cinnamon

- 4 cups apples, diced

Directions:

1. Preheat the oven to 375°F and oil a loaf pan with non-stick spray or your choice of oil.
2. Beat the eggs in a mixing bowl and stir until completely smooth.
3. Add the honey, oil, applesauce, cinnamon, vanilla, nutmeg, baking powder, baking soda, and salt. Whisk until completely combined and smooth.
4. Add the flour into the bowl and whisk to combine, making sure not to over-mix. Simply stir it enough to incorporate the flour.
5. Add the apples to the batter and mix again to combine.
6. Pour the batter into the loaf pan and smooth the top with your spatula.
7. Bake for 20 minutes, or until an inserted toothpick in the center comes out clean.
8. Let stand for 10 minutes, and then transfer the loaf to a cooling rack to cool completely.
9. Slice into 10 pieces and serve!

Nutrition:

- Calories: 210
- Carbohydrates: 41 g
- Fats: 5 g
- Protein: 5 g

43. Zucchini Chips

Preparation Time: 10 minutes

Cooking Time: 12 minutes

Servings: 4

Ingredients:

- 1 zucchini, thinly sliced
- A pinch of sea salt
- Black pepper to taste
- 1 teaspoon thyme, dried
- 1 egg
- 1 teaspoon garlic powder
- 1 cup almond flour

Directions:

1. In a bowl, whisk the egg with a pinch of salt.
2. Put the flour in another bowl and mix it with thyme, black pepper, and garlic powder.
3. Dredge zucchini slices in the egg mixture and then in flour.
4. Arrange chips on a lined baking sheet, place in the oven at 450°F and bake for 6 minutes on each side.
5. Serve the zucchini chips as a snack. Enjoy.

Nutrition:

- Calories: 106
- **Fat:** 8.2 g
- Carbohydrates: 5.2 g
- Protein: 5.1 g
- **Fiber:** 2.1 g

44. Coconut Protein Balls

Preparation Time: 20 minutes

Cooking Time: 0 minutes

Servings: 27

Ingredients:

- ¼ cup dark chocolate chips
- ½ cup coconut flakes, unsweetened
- ½ cup water
- 1 ½ cup almonds, raw and unsalted
- 2 tablespoons cocoa powder, unsweetened
- 3 cups Medjool dates, pitted

- 4 scoops whey protein powder, unsweetened

Directions:

1. Blend almonds in a food processor until flour is formed. Add the water and dates to the flour and continue to process until fully combined. You may need to stop intermittently to scrape down the sides of the bowl.
2. Add cocoa and protein to the processor and continue to process until well combined. You may need to stop intermittently to scrape down the sides of the bowl.
3. Pull the blade out of the processor (carefully!) and use your spatula to gather all of the dough in one place inside the processor container.
4. On a plate or in a large, shallow dish, spread the coconut flakes.
5. Scoop out a little bit of the dough at a time using a spoon, and roll it into balls, then roll each one in the coconut flakes and chocolate chips.
6. Refrigerate for at least 30 minutes before enjoying.

Nutrition:

- Calories: 108
- Carbohydrates: 16 g
- Fats: 4 g
- Protein: 5 g

45. Pepperoni Bites

Preparation Time: 5 minutes

Cooking Time: 10 minutes

Servings: 24 pieces

Ingredients:

- 1/3 cup tomatoes, chopped
- ½ cup bell peppers, mixed and chopped
- 24 pepperoni slices
- ½ cup tomato sauce
- 4 ounces almond cheese, cubed
- 2 tablespoons basil, chopped
- Black pepper to taste

Directions:

1. Divide the pepperoni slices into a muffin tray.
2. Divide the tomato and bell pepper pieces into the pepperoni cups.
3. Also divide the tomato sauce, basil, and almond cheese cubes, sprinkle black pepper at the end, place the cups in the oven at 400°F and bake for 10 minutes.
4. Arrange the pepperoni bites on a platter and serve.

Nutrition:

- Calories: 59
- Fat: 4.5 g
- Fiber: 0.1 g
- Carbohydrates: 2 g
- Protein: 2.5 g

46. Blueberry Muffins

Preparation Time: 5 minutes

Cooking Time: 25 minutes

Servings: 12

Ingredients:

- ½ teaspoon baking soda
- ¼ cup vegetable oil
- ¼ teaspoon salt
- 1 ½ cup blueberries, frozen
- 1 cup applesauce, unsweetened
- 1 teaspoon vanilla extract
- 1/3 cup honey
- 2 cup whole wheat flour
- 1 teaspoon cinnamon
- 2 large eggs, beaten

- 2 teaspoons baking powder

Directions:

Preheat the oven to 350°F and line a muffin tin with paper liners.

Combine the eggs, applesauce, honey, oil, vanilla extract, cinnamon, baking soda, salt, and baking powder in a bowl. Whisk until completely combined, ensuring that there are no lumps of baking powder or soda.

Add flour to the batter and whisk until just combined.

Add blueberries and mix.

Fill the muffin tins and bake for 22–25 minutes or until a toothpick inserted in the middle of the middlemost muffin becomes clean.

Let cool for 30 minutes before transferring to a cooling rack to cool completely.

1. Serve and enjoy!

Nutrition:

- Calories: 329
- Carbohydrates: 40 g
- Fats: 14 g
- Protein: 14 g

47. Cauliflower Fried Rice

Preparation Time: 10 minutes

Cooking Time: 10 minutes

Servings: 5

Ingredients:

- 1 head cauliflower, halved
- 2 tablespoons sesame oil
- 2 onions, chopped
- 1 Egg, beaten
- 5 tablespoons coconut aminos
- 1 cup water
- Salt and pepper, to taste

Directions:

1. Place a steam rack in the Instant Pot and add a cup of water.

2. Place the cauliflower florets on the steam rack.

3. Set the lid in place and the vent to point to "Sealing."

4. Press the "Steam" button and adjust the time to 7 minutes.

5. Release the pressure quickly.

6. In a food processor, add in cauliflower florets and pulse until grainy in texture.

7. Sauté the oil.

8. Stir in the onions until fragrant.

9. Stir in the egg and break it up into small pieces.

10. Add the cauliflower rice and season with coconut aminos.

11. Add in more pepper and salt if desired.

Nutrition:

- Calories: 108
- Carbohydrates: 4.3 g
- Protein: 3.4 g
- Fat: 8.2 g

48. Protein Bars

Preparation Time: 10 minutes

Cooking Time: 30 minutes

Servings: 12

Ingredients:

For the Bars

- 1/3 cup coconut oil
- 1/3 cup creamy peanut butter, unsalted
- 1/3 cup almond meal
- ½ cup milk of your choice, unsweetened
- 1 ½ cup protein powder

For the Topping

- 2 tablespoons chocolate chips
- 1 tablespoon coconut oil
- 3 tablespoons almonds, chopped

Directions:

In a microwave-safe bowl, combine peanut butter, milk and all but one tablespoon of coconut oil. Heat for 30-second intervals, stirring in between, until completely smooth.

Mix almond meal and protein powder into the bowl and combine well until a crumbly dough is combined.

Line a baking dish with parchment paper and flatten the dough into it until an even layer is formed.

In a small, microwave-safe bowl, put the chocolate chips and 1 tablespoon of coconut oil and heat for 30-second intervals, while stirring in between until completely smooth.

Pour the mixture of chocolate over the bars and spread it evenly. Sprinkle the almonds on top and then freeze the bars for about 20 minutes, or refrigerate them for about an hour.

1. Cut into 12 evenly-shaped bars and enjoy!

Nutrition:

- Calories: 186
- Carbohydrates: 7 g
- Fat: 14 g
- Protein: 8 g

49. Almond Bites

Preparation Time: 10 minutes

Cooking Time: 14 minutes

Servings: 5

Ingredients:

- 1 cup almond flour
- ¼ cup almond milk
- 1 egg, whisked
- 2 tablespoons butter
- 1 tablespoon coconut flakes
- ½ teaspoon baking powder
- ½ teaspoon apple cider vinegar
- ½ teaspoon vanilla extract

Directions:

1. Mix up together the whisked egg, almond milk, apple cider vinegar, baking powder, vanilla extract, and butter.
2. Stir the mixture and add almond flour and coconut flakes. Knead the dough.
3. If the dough is sticky, add more almond flour. Make the medium balls from the dough and place them on the rack of Ninja Foodi.
4. Press them gently with the hand palm. Lower the air fryer lid and cook the dessert for 12 minutes at 360°F.
5. Check if the dessert is cooked; and cook for 2 minutes more for a crunchy crust.

Nutrition:

- Calories: 118
- Fats: 11.5 g
- Carbohydrates: 2.4 g
- Protein: 2.7 g

50. Summer Swiss Chard

Preparation Time: 5 minutes

Cooking Time: 15 minutes

Servings: 4

Ingredients:

- 1 pound Swiss chard
- 3 tablespoons olive oil
- 1 cup onion, diced
- A pinch salt
- ½ teaspoon oregano
- 3 tablespoons red-wine vinegar
- Salt and pepper to taste

Directions:

1. Chop the chard and set aside.

2. Heat the olive oil in a skillet over medium heat.

3. Add the diced onion, a pinch of salt, and oregano and cook until the onions are tender.

4. Add the chopped chard and sauté for a few minutes and then remove from heat.

5. Stir in the vinegar and season with salt and pepper.

Nutrition:

- Calories: 132
- Fat: 11 g
- Protein: 3 g
- Carbohydrates: 8 g

51. Healthy Salmon Burgers

Preparation Time: 10 minutes

Cooking Time: 10 minutes

Servings: 6

Ingredients:

- 2 salmon fillets
- 2 eggs
- ½ cup chopped onions
- 1 tablespoon mayonnaise
- 1 cup gluten-free bread crumbs
- 2 teaspoons lemon juice
- ¼ teaspoon garlic salt
- 1 tablespoon chopped fresh parsley
- 3 tablespoons olive oil
- Salt and pepper to taste

Directions:

1. Season the salmon using salt and pepper.
2. In a skillet add ½ tablespoon of oil and heat it over medium heat.
3. Fry the salmon for 2 minutes on both sides.
4. Let it cool down completely.
5. Remove the bones and mash it finely.
6. Transfer the salmon to a bowl. Add the onion, garlic salt, parsley, lemon juice, bread crumbs, mayo, and eggs.
7. Mix well and create burger patties using your hands.
8. Let it refrigerate for 30 minutes.
9. In a skillet heat the remaining oil.
10. Fry the patties golden brown.
11. Make sure to fry in batches.
12. Serve warm.

Nutrition:

- Calories: 254
- Fats: 20 g
- Protein: 15 g
- Carbohydrates: 8 g

52. Roasted Brussels Sprouts with Pecans and Gorgonzola

Preparation Time: 10 minutes

Cooking Time: 35 minutes

Servings: 4

Ingredients:

- 1 pound Brussels sprouts, fresh
- ¼ cup pecans, chopped
- 1 tablespoon olive oil
- Extra-virgin olive oil to oil the baking tray
- Pepper and salt to taste
- ¼ cup Gorgonzola cheese (If you prefer not to use the Gorgonzola cheese, you can toss the Brussels sprouts when hot, with 2 tablespoons of butter instead.)

Directions:

1. Preheat the oven to 350°F or 175°C.
2. Rub a large pan or any vessel you wish to use with a little bit of olive oil. You can use a paper towel or a pastry brush.
3. Cut off the ends of the Brussels sprouts if you need to and then cut them in a lengthwise direction into halves. (Don't be afraid if a few of the leaves come off, some may become deliciously crunchy during cooking.)
4. Chop up all of the pecans using a knife and then measure them for the amount.
5. Put your Brussels sprouts as well as the sliced pecans inside a bowl, and cover them all with some olive oil, pepper, and salt (be generous).
6. Arrange all of your pecans and Brussels sprouts onto your roasting pan in a single layer.
7. Roast this for 30 to 35 minutes, or when they become tender and can be pierced with a fork easily. Stir during cooking if you wish to get a more even browning.
8. Once cooked, toss them with the Gorgonzola Cheese (or butter) before you serve them. Serve them hot.

Nutrition:

- Calories: 149
- **Fat:** 11 g
- Carbohydrates: 10 g
- Fiber: 4 g
- Protein: 5 g

53. Artichoke Petals Bites

Preparation Time: 10 minutes

Cooking Time: 10 minutes

Servings: 8

Ingredients:

- 8 ounces artichoke petals, boiled, drained, without salt
- ½ cup almond flour
- 4 ounces Parmesan, grated
- 2 tablespoons almond butter, melted

Directions:

1. In the mixing bowl, mix up together almond flour and grated Parmesan.
2. Preheat the oven to 355°F.
3. Dip the artichoke petals in the almond butter and then coat in the almond flour mixture.
4. Place them in the tray.
5. Transfer the tray to the preheated oven and cook the petals for 10 minutes.
6. Chill the cooked petal bites a little before serving.

Nutrition:

- Calories: 93
- Protein: 6.54 g
- **Fat:** 3.72 g
- Carbohydrates: 9.08 g

54. Stuffed Beef Loin in Sticky Sauce

Preparation Time: 15 minutes

Cooking Time: 40 minutes

Servings: 4

Ingredients:

- 1 tablespoon Erythritol
- 1 tablespoon lemon juice
- 4 tablespoons water
- 1 tablespoon butter
- ½ teaspoon tomato sauce
- ¼ teaspoon dried rosemary
- 9 ounces beef loin
- 3 ounces celery root, grated
- 3 ounces bacon, sliced
- 1 tablespoon walnuts, chopped
- ¾ teaspoon garlic, diced
- 2 teaspoons butter
- 1 tablespoon olive oil
- 1 teaspoon salt
- ½ cup water

Directions:

1. Cut the beef loin into the layer and spread it with the dried rosemary, butter, and salt. Then place over the beef loin: grated celery root, sliced bacon, walnuts, and diced garlic.
2. Roll the beef loin and brush it with olive oil. Secure the meat with the help of the toothpicks. Place it in the tray and add a ½ cup of water.
3. Cook the meat in the preheated to 365°F oven for 40 minutes.
4. Meanwhile, make the sticky sauce:
5. Mix up together Erythritol, lemon juice, 4 tablespoons of water, and butter.
6. Preheat the mixture until it starts to boil. Then add the tomato sauce and whisk it well.
7. Bring the sauce to a boil and remove it from the heat.
8. When the beef loin is cooked, remove it from the oven and brush it with the cooked sticky sauce very generously.
9. Slice the beef roll and sprinkle with the remaining sauce.

Nutrition:

- Calories: 321
- **Protein:** 18.35 g

- **Fat:** 26.68 g
- Carbohydrates: 2.75 g

55. Eggplant Fries

Preparation Time: 10 minutes

Cooking Time: 15 minutes

Servings: 8

Ingredients:

- 2 eggs
- 2 cups almond flour
- 2 tablespoons coconut oil, spray
- 2 eggplants, peeled and cut thinly
- Salt and pepper, to taste

Directions:

1. Preheat your oven to 400°F.
2. Take a bowl and mix with flour and salt and black pepper in it.
3. Take another bowl and beat eggs until frothy.
4. Dip the eggplant pieces into eggs.
5. Then coat them with the flour mixture.
6. Add another layer of flour and egg.
7. Then, take a baking sheet and grease with coconut oil on top.
8. Bake for about 15 minutes.
9. Serve and enjoy.

Nutrition:

- Calories: 212
- **Fat:** 15.8 g
- Carbohydrates: 12.1 g
- Protein: 8.6 g

56. Parmesan Crisps

Preparation Time: 5 minutes

Cooking Time: 25 minutes

Servings: 8

Ingredients:

- 1 teaspoon butter
- 8 ounces Parmesan cheese, full fat and shredded

Directions:

1. Preheat your oven to 400°F.
2. Put parchment paper on a baking sheet and grease with butter.
3. Spoon Parmesan into 8 mounds, spreading them apart evenly.
4. Flatten them.
5. Bake for 5 minutes until browned.
6. Let them cool.
7. Serve and enjoy.

Nutrition:

- Calories: 133
- **Fat:** 11 g
- Carbohydrates: 1 g
- Protein: 11 g

57. Baked Fennel

Preparation Time: 10 minutes

Cooking Time: 45 minutes

Servings: 6

Ingredients:

- 3 fennel bulbs
- 1 cup chicken broth
- ¼ cup Gorgonzola cheese, crumbled
- ¼ cup panko bread crumbs
- Salt and pepper to taste

Directions:

Cut the fennel bulbs in half lengthwise through the root end.

Put the fennel cut-side down in a skillet and add the chicken broth. Cover and simmer for 20 minutes.

Preheat the oven to 375°F. Place the cooked fennel bulbs in a baking dish, cut-sides up.

Mix the Gorgonzola with the bread crumbs and divide the mixture evenly on the top of each fennel bulb.

Bake for 25 minutes, season with salt and pepper and serve hot.

Nutrition:

- Calories: 75
- **Fat:** 2 g
- Protein: 3 g
- Carbohydrates: 12 g

58. Pumpkin Pie

Preparation Time: 10 minutes

Cooking Time: 25 minutes

Servings: 6

Ingredients:

- 1 cup coconut flour
- ¼ cup heavy cream
- 1 egg, whisked
- 1 tablespoon butter
- 2 tablespoons liquid stevia
- 1 tablespoon pumpkin puree
- 1 teaspoon apple cider vinegar
- 1 teaspoon Pumpkin spices
- ½ teaspoon baking powder

Directions:

1. Melt the butter and combine it together with the heavy cream, apple cider vinegar, liquid stevia, egg, and baking powder.
2. Add pumpkin puree and coconut flour. Now, add pumpkin spices and stir the batter until smooth.
3. Pour the batter into the Ninja Foodi basket and lower the air fryer lid.
4. Set the "Bake" mode 360°F. Cook the pie for 25 minutes. When the time is over, let the pie chill until it is room temperature.

Nutrition:

- Calories: 127
- **Fat:** 6.6 g
- Carbohydrates: 14.2 g
- Protein: 3.8 g

59. Brownie Batter

Preparation Time: 5 minutes

Cooking Time: 4 minutes

Servings: 5

Ingredients:

- 1 ounce dark chocolate
- ¼ cup heavy cream
- 1/3 cup almond flour
- 1 tablespoon Erythritol
- 3 tablespoons cocoa powder
- 3 tablespoons butter
- ½ teaspoon vanilla extract

Directions:

1. Place the almond flour in the springform pan and flatten to make the layer. Then place the springform pan in the pot and lower the air fryer lid.
2. Cook the almond flour for 3 minutes at 400°F or until the almond flour gets a golden color.
3. Meanwhile, combine together cocoa powder and heavy cream; whisk the heavy cream until smooth.
4. Add vanilla extract and Erythritol. Remove the almond flour from Ninja Foodi and chill well.
5. Toss butter and dark chocolate in the pot and preheat for 1 minute on "Sauté" mode.
6. When the butter is soft; add it to the heavy cream mixture. Then add chocolate and almond flour. Stir the mass until homogenous and serve!

Nutrition:

- Calories: 159
- **Fats:** 14.9 g
- Carbohydrates: 9 g
- Protein: 2.5 g

60. Meatloaf

Preparation Time: 10 minutes

Cooking Time: 40 minutes

Servings: 9

Ingredients:

- 2 cups ground beef
- 1 cup ground chicken
- 2 eggs
- 1 tablespoon salt
- 1 teaspoon ground black pepper
- ½ teaspoon paprika
- 1 tablespoon butter
- 1 teaspoon cilantro
- 1 tablespoon basil
- ¼ cup fresh dill
- 1 cup breadcrumbs

Directions:

1. Combine the chicken with the ground beef in a mixing bowl.
2. Add egg, salt, ground black pepper, paprika, butter, cilantro, and basil.
3. Chop the dill and add it to the ground meat mixture and stir using your hand.
4. Place the meat mixture on an aluminum foil and add breadcrumbs before wrapping it.
5. Place it in a pressure cooker and close its lid. Cook the dish on "Sauté" mode and cook for 40 minutes.
6. When the cooking time ends, remove your meatloaf from the cooker and allow it to cool.
7. Unwrap the foil, slice it, and serve.

Nutrition:

- Calories: 173
- **Fats:** 11.5 g
- Carbohydrates: 0.81 g
- Protein: 16 g

61. Broccoli Rabe with Lemon and Cheese

Preparation Time: 5 minutes

Cooking Time: 15 minutes

Servings: 4

Ingredients:

- 1 quart water
- 1 teaspoon salt
- ½ cup broccoli rabe, trimmed
- 2 tablespoons olive oil
- 2 cloves garlic, chopped
- 1 tablespoon lemon juice
- Salt and pepper to taste
- 2 tablespoons Parmesan cheese

Directions:

Boil water; add salt and broccoli rabe. On low heat, simmer for about 8 minutes. Drain and shock under cold water and dry on paper towels.

Heat olive oil over medium-low heat and sauté the garlic for 5 minutes. Cut the broccoli rabe stems into 2 pieces and add to the garlic and olive oil. Sprinkle with lemon juice, salt, and pepper. Serve the Parmesan cheese at the table.

Nutrition:

Calories: 81

Fat: 8 g

Protein: 2 g

Carbohydrates: 2 g

62. Dried Tomatoes

Preparation Time: 5 minutes

Cooking Time: 8 hours

Servings: 8

Ingredients:

- 5 medium tomatoes
- 1 tablespoon basil
- 1 teaspoon cilantro
- 1 tablespoon onion powder
- 5 tablespoons organic olive oil
- 1 teaspoon paprika

Directions:

1. Wash the tomatoes and slice them.
2. Combine cilantro with basil, onion powder, and paprika. Stir well.
3. Place the sliced tomatoes in the pressure cooker and add the spice mixture.
4. Add organic olive oil and close the lid.
5. Cook the dish on "Slow" mode for 8 hours.
6. When the cooking time ends, the tomatoes should be semi-dry. Remove them from the pressure cooker.
7. Serve your dried tomatoes warm.

Nutrition:

- Calories: 92
- Fats: 8.6 g
- Proteins: 1 g
- Carbohydrates: 3.84 g

CHAPTER 12.

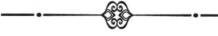

MAIN COURSE: 25 RECIPES

63. Meaty Spaghetti Squash

Preparation Time: 10 minutes

Cooking Time: 50 minutes

Servings: 6

Ingredients:

- 1 egg
- 1 teaspoon oregano dried
- 1 teaspoon basil dried
- ¼ cup grated Parmesan cheese
- ½ teaspoon salt
- 4 cups minced beef
- 1 teaspoon Worcestershire sauce.
- 3 cups marinara sauce low carb
- 2 cups mozzarella cheese shredded
- 4 cups low-carb cooked spaghetti squash

Directions:

1. Heat your oven in advance at 250°C.
2. Take a mixing container and in it mix the minced beef, Worcestershire sauce, basil dried, oregano dried, egg, salt, and Parmesan cheese grated.
3. Take small scoops of the mix and make balls of meat taking care because they will be very soft.
4. Take a sheet used for baking and coat its bottom with a quarter cup of the marinara sauce. Arrange the balls of meat you have prepared at the top and then pour the remaining marinara sauce at the top coating all of them.
5. Place the sheet for baking in the oven you had heated in advance and let the balls of meat bake for ½ hour until well cooked.

6. After half an hour, sprinkle the shredded mozzarella cheese on top of the baked balls of meat and then replace it in the oven for the cheese to melt for about 3 minutes.

7. When all the cheese has melted, take them out of the oven and allow them to get cold completely before serving.

8. Take a plate and in it, place the spaghetti squash and scoops of the baked balls of meat and enjoy.

Nutrition:

- Calories: 210 g
- Fat: 12 g
- Fiber: 2 g
- Carbohydrates: 8 g
- Protein: 6 g

64. Cajun Pork Sliders

Preparation Time: 10 minutes

Cooking Time: 45 minutes

Servings: 4

Ingredients:

- 4 low-carb bread slices
- 14 ounces pork loin
- 2 tablespoons Cajun spices
- 1 tablespoon olive oil
- 1/3 cup water
- 1 teaspoon of tomato sauce

Directions:

1. Rub the pork loin with Cajun spices and place in the skillet.
2. Add olive oil and roast it over high heat for 5 minutes from each side.
3. After this, transfer the meat to the saucepan, add tomato sauce and water.
4. Stir gently and close the lid.
5. Simmer the meat for 35 minutes.
6. Slice the cooked pork loin.
7. Place the pork sliders over the bread slices and transfer them to the serving plates.

Nutrition:

- Calories: 382
- **Fat:** 22.4
- Fiber: 4.5
- Carbohydrates: 2.4
- Protein: 38.9

65. Sausage Casserole

Preparation Time: 10 minutes

Cooking Time: 35 minutes

Servings: 6

Ingredients:

- 2 jalapeno peppers, sliced
- 5 ounces Cheddar cheese, shredded
- 9 ounces sausages, chopped
- 1 tablespoon olive oil
- ½ cup spinach, chopped
- ½ cup heavy cream
- ½ teaspoon salt

Directions:

1. Brush the casserole mold with the olive oil from inside.
2. Then put the chopped sausages in the casserole mold in one layer.
3. Add chopped spinach and sprinkle it with salt.
4. After this, add sliced jalapeno pepper.
5. Then make the layer of shredded Cheddar cheese.
6. Pour the heavy cream over the cheese.
7. Preheat the oven to 355°F.
8. Transfer the casserole to the oven and cook it for 35 minutes.
9. Use the kitchen torch to make the crunchy cheese crust of the casserole.

Nutrition:

- Calories: 296
- Fat: 26
- Fiber: 0.3
- Carbohydrates: 1
- Protein: 14.5

66. Beef Stroganoff

Preparation Time: 10 minutes

Cooking Time: 30 minutes

Servings: 6

Ingredients:

- 1 (10-ounce) package of egg noodles, cooked according to the package instructions.
- 2 pounds of beef steak, sliced into thin strips
- 4 tablespoons butter
- 2 cups brown or cremini mushrooms, sliced
- 1 large white or yellow onion, sliced
- 2 medium garlic cloves, minced
- ½ cup sour cream
- ¼ cup flour
- 2 teaspoons Worcestershire sauce
- 1 teaspoon Dijon mustard
- 1 teaspoon smoked paprika or regular paprika
- 3 cups homemade low-sodium beef stock
- ½ teaspoon fine sea salt
- ½ teaspoon freshly cracked black pepper

Direction:

1. In a large skillet over medium-high heat, add 2 tablespoons of butter.
2. Add the beef strips and cook until brown. Remove and set aside.
3. Add the remaining 2 tablespoons of butter to the skillet along with the sliced mushrooms, chopped onion, salt, pepper, and minced garlic. Sauté until the vegetables have softened, stirring occasionally.
4. Sprinkle ¼ cup of flour over the vegetables and cook for another minute, stirring occasionally.
5. Lower the heat and stir in the beef stock while whisking constantly. Allow simmering until thickens.
6. Stir in the Worcestershire sauce, Dijon mustard, smoked paprika, and sour cream until well combined.
7. Stir in the beef strips and simmer for another 5 minutes.
8. Serve over egg noodles.

Nutrition:

- Calories: 497
- Fat: 22 g
- Fiber: 2 g
- Carbohydrates: 19 g
- Protein: 49 g

67. Tasteful Beef Burrito Skillet

Preparation Time: 10 minutes

Cooking Time: 20 minutes

Servings: 6

Ingredients:

- 1 pound lean grass-fed ground beef
- 1 (1-ounce) package of taco seasoning mix
- 1 cup mild chunky salsa
- 4 flour tortillas, sliced into strips
- 1 (15-ounce) can of black beans, drained and rinsed
- 1 cup water
- 1 cup shredded Mexican blend cheese
- ½ cup sour cream
- ¼ cup green onions, sliced

Directions:

1. In a large non-stick skillet over medium-high heat, add the ground beef. Cook until brown, stirring occasionally. Drain the excess liquid.
2. Add the taco seasoning mix, mild chunky salsa, and black beans and 1 cup of water. Reduce the heat.
3. Stir in the tortilla strips and top with the shredded Mexican blend cheese. Remove from the heat and allow the cheese to melt.
4. Top with sour cream and sprinkle with sliced green onions
5. Serve and enjoy!

Nutrition:

- Calories: 384
- Fat: 21 g
- Fiber: 7 g
- Carbohydrates: 28 g
- Protein: 24 g

68. No Cheese Quesadillas

Preparation Time: 10 minutes

Cooking Time: 30 minutes

Servings: 3

Ingredients:

- Extra chunky salsa, as required
- 12 yellow no oil corn tortillas
- 2 medium onions, chopped
- 1 small yellow bell pepper, chopped
- 1 small green bell pepper, chopped
- 1 small red bell pepper, chopped
- 1 ½ cup no oil refried pinto beans
- Chili powder, to taste

Directions:

1. Place a tortilla on your countertop. Spread 4 tablespoons refried beans over it.
2. Sprinkle a little of onions, bell peppers, and chili powder over it.
3. Cover with another tortilla.
4. Place a non-stick pan over medium heat. Carefully lift the quesadilla and place it on the pan. Cook until the underside is crisp. Flip sides and cook the other side until crisp.
5. Repeat steps 1–4 to make the remaining quesadillas.
6. Cut each into 4 wedges and serve with salsa.

Nutrition:

- Calories: 191
- Fat: 9 g
- Fiber: 2 g
- Carbohydrates: 8 g
- Protein: 20 g

69. Pea and Farro Stir-Fry

Preparation Time: 10 minutes

Cooking Time: 30 minutes

Servings: 3

Ingredients:

- ½ cup fresh basil, torn
- ½ teaspoon paprika
- 2 cups fresh or frozen peas, thaw if frozen
- 1 1/3 cup cooked farro
- Pepper to taste
- Salt to taste
- 4 cloves garlic, minced
- 1 medium sweet onion, thinly sliced
- 4 large eggs, beaten
- 4 teaspoons olive oil, divided

Directions:

1. Place a large cast-iron skillet over medium-high heat. Add 2 teaspoons of oil. When the oil is heated, crack the eggs and stir constantly until scrambled and cooked.
2. Add garlic, pepper, and salt and sauté until aromatic.
3. Stir in the rest of the ingredients and heat thoroughly.

Nutrition:

- Calories: 191
- Fat: 9 g
- Fiber: 2 g
- Carbohydrates: 8 g
- Protein: 20 g

70. Lemon Baked Salmon

Preparation Time: 5 minutes

Cooking Time: 20 minutes

Servings: 2

Ingredients:

- 12 ounces filets of salmon
- 2 lemons, sliced thinly
- 2 tablespoons olive oil
- Salt and black pepper, to taste
- 3 sprigs thyme

Directions:

1. Preheat the oven to 350°F.
2. Place half the sliced lemons on the bottom of a baking dish.
3. Place the fillets over the lemons and cover with the remaining lemon slices and thyme.
4. Drizzle olive oil over the dish and cook for 20 minutes.
5. Season with salt and pepper.

Nutrition:

- Calories: 571
- Fat: 44 g
- Fiber: 2 g
- Carbohydrates: 2 g
- Protein: 42 g

71. Seafood Casserole

Preparation Time: 30 minutes

Cooking Time: 35 minutes

Servings: 6

Ingredients:

Poached Seafood

- 1 cup dry white wine
- 1 cup water
- 2 small bay leaves, whole
- ½ teaspoon old bay seasoning
- 1 ounce shrimp, thawed, peeled and deveined
- 12 ounces cod, diced

Vegetables

- 2 stalks celery, diced
- 2 tablespoons butter
- 2 medium leeks, white part only, sliced
- Sea salt, to taste

Sauce

- ½ teaspoon xanthan gum
- 1 cup heavy whipping cream
- 1 tablespoon butter
- ¼ teaspoon sea salt

Topping

- 1 tablespoon butter
- 4 ounces Parmesan cheese, shredded
- 2 teaspoons old bay seasoning
- ¼ cup almond flour
- 1 tablespoon fresh parsley, chopped

Direction:

1. Set the oven's temperature at 400°F to preheat.
2. Take a large-sized saucepan and place it over medium-high heat.
3. Add dry white wine, bay leaves, water, and ½ teaspoon old bay to the saucepan.
4. Cook the mixture for 3 minutes on a simmer.
5. Add shrimp to the wine mixture and cook until the shrimp changes color.

6. Remove the shrimp from the poaching liquid using a slotted spoon and transfer it to a plate.

7. Add the cod to the poaching liquid and cook until the fish turns white.

8. Remove the codfish from the liquid and keep it aside on a plate.

9. Cook the poaching liquid until it is reduced to 1 cup.

10. Take a Dutch oven and place it over medium-high heat.

11. Add 2 tablespoons butter to the Dutch oven and melt it.

12. Stir in leeks and celery then stir-fry until soft.

13. Season the vegetables with sea salt, and then remove them from heat.

14. Spread the vegetables in a casserole dish, then toss in the seafood.

15. Add the sauce ingredients to the same Dutch oven and cook, stirring until it thickens.

16. Pour the sauce over the seafood in the casserole dish.

17. Prepare the topping by blending almond flour with 1 tablespoon butter, 2 teaspoons old bay, and Parmesan cheese.

18. Spread this crumble over the seafood mixture and then bake for 20 minutes in the oven.

19. Serve warm and fresh.

Nutrition:

- Calories: 292
- Total Fat: 12.9 g
- Saturated Fat: 7.7 g
- Carbohydrates: 3.6 g
- Dietary Fiber: 0.1 g
- **Sugars**: 0.5 g
- Protein: 32.5 g

72. **Shrimp Scampi**

Preparation Time: 20 minutes

Cooking Time: 12 minutes

Servings: 6

Ingredients:

- 1 ¼ pound shrimp, peeled and deveined
- 4 tablespoons butter
- 3 garlic cloves, roughly chopped
- ¼ cup Chardonnay
- ¼ cup lemon juice
- ¼ teaspoon red pepper flakes
- ¼ cup parsley, chopped
- 2 scallions, sliced
- ½ cup shredded Parmesan cheese
- Salt and black pepper, to taste
- 1 ounce cherry tomatoes, halved

Directions:

1. Peel and devein the shrimp and keep them ready aside.
2. Finely chop the parsley and garlic.
3. Take a large-sized sauté pan and place it over medium heat.
4. Add butter to the pan and heat it to melt.
5. Stir in garlic and cherry tomatoes and sauté until soft.
6. Toss in shrimp and stir-fry until they turn pink.
7. Flip the shrimp, add the scallions and season with red pepper flakes.
8. Add lemon juice and wine, and then cook until the liquid is reduced.
9. Remove the shrimp from heat and add parsley.
10. Garnish with Parmesan and serve warm.

Nutrition:

- Calories: 210
- Total Fat: 10 g
- Saturated Fat: 5.8 g
- Carbohydrates: 5.5 g
- Dietary Fiber: 0.9 g
- **Sugars:** 2.6 g
- Protein: 23.2 g

73. Easy Blackened Shrimp

Preparation Time: 10 minutes

Cooking Time: 6 minutes

Servings: 2

Ingredients:

- ½ pound shrimp, peeled and deveined
- 2 tablespoons blackened seasoning
- 1 teaspoon olive oil
- Juice of 1 lemon

Directions:

1. Toss all ingredients (except oil) together until shrimp are well coated.
2. In a non-stick skillet, heat the oil to medium-high heat.
3. Add shrimp and cook 2–3 minutes per side.
4. Serve immediately.

Nutrition:

- Calories: 152
- Fat: 4 g
- Fiber: 1 g
- Carbohydrates: 8 g
- Protein: 24 g

74. BBQ Pork Tenders

Preparation Time: 15 minutes

Cooking Time: 7 minutes

Servings: 4

Ingredients:

- 1 teaspoon Erythritol
- 3 tablespoons ground paprika
- 1 teaspoon ground black pepper
- 1 teaspoon salt
- ½ teaspoon chili powder
- ¼ teaspoon cayenne pepper
- 1 teaspoon garlic powder
- 14 ounces pork loin
- 1 tablespoon olive oil
- 1 tablespoon almond butter

Directions:

1. Make the BBQ mix: in the shallow bowl, mix up together ground paprika, Erythritol, ground black pepper, salt, chili powder, cayenne pepper, and garlic powder.
2. Cut the pork loin into the tenders.
3. Rub every pork loin with BBQ mix and sprinkle with olive oil.
4. Leave the meat to marinate for at least 15 minutes.
5. After this, place almond butter in the skillet and melt it.
6. Place the pork tenders in the almond butter and cook them for 5 minutes.
7. Then flip the meat onto another side and cook for 2 minutes more. The time of cooking depends on the meat thickness.

Nutrition:

- Calories: 315
- Fat: 20.3
- Fiber: 2.7
- Carbohydrates: 4.7
- Protein: 29

75. Pan-fried Cod

Preparation Time: 5 minutes

Cooking Time: 10 minutes

Servings: 2

Ingredients:

- 12 ounces cod fillet
- 1 tablespoon scallions, chopped
- 1 tablespoon butter
- 1 tablespoon coconut oil
- 1 teaspoon garlic, diced
- 1 teaspoon cumin seeds
- 1 teaspoon coriander seeds
- 1 teaspoon salt

Directions:

1. Place butter and coconut oil in the skillet and melt them.
2. Add garlic, cumin, scallions and coriander seeds.
3. Rub the fish fillet with salt and place it in the skillet.
4. Fry the fish for 2 minutes from each side or until it is light brown.
5. Transfer the cooked cod fillet to the plate and cut into 2 servings.

Nutrition:

- Calories: 253
- Fat: 14.3
- Fiber: 0.2
- Carbohydrates: 1.2
- Protein: 30.8

76. Grilled Shrimp Easy Seasoning

Preparation Time: 5 minutes

Cooking Time: 5 minutes

Servings: 4

Ingredients:

Shrimp Seasoning

- 1 teaspoon garlic powder
- 1 teaspoon kosher salt
- 1 teaspoon Italian seasoning
- ¼ teaspoon cayenne pepper

Grilling

- 2 tablespoons olive oil
- 1 tablespoon lemon juice
- 1 pound jumbo shrimp, peeled, deveined
- Ghee for the grill

Directions:

1. Preheat the grill pan over high heat.
2. In a mixing bowl, stir together the seasoning ingredients.
3. Drizzle in the lemon juice and olive oil and stir.
4. Add the shrimp and toss to coat.
5. Brush the grill pan with ghee.
6. Grill the shrimp until pink, about 2–3 minutes per side.
7. Serve immediately.

Nutrition:

- Calories: 101
- Fat: 3 g
- Fiber: 1 g
- Carbohydrates: 1 g
- Protein: 28 g

77. Butter Chicken

Preparation Time: 5 minutes

Cooking Time: 30 minutes

Servings: 4

Ingredients:

- ¼ cup butter
- 2 cups mushrooms, sliced
- 4 large chicken thighs
- ½ teaspoon onion powder
- ½ teaspoon garlic powder
- 1 teaspoon kosher salt
- ¼ teaspoon black pepper
- ½ cup water
- 1 teaspoon Dijon mustard
- 1 tablespoon fresh tarragon, chopped

Directions:

1. Season the chicken thighs with onion powder, garlic powder, salt, and pepper.
2. In a sauté pan, melt 1 tablespoon of butter.
3. Sear the chicken thighs for about 3 to 4 minutes per side, or until both sides are golden brown. Remove the thighs from the pan.
4. Add the remaining 3 tablespoons of butter to the pan and melt.
5. Add the mushrooms and cook for 4 to 5 minutes or until golden brown. Stirring as little as possible.
6. Add the Dijon mustard and water to the pan. Stir to deglaze.
7. Place the chicken thighs back in the pan with the skin side up.
8. Cover and simmer for 15 minutes.
9. Stir in the fresh herbs. Let sit for 5 minutes and serve.

Nutrition:

- Calories: 414
- Fat: 9 g
- Fiber: 2 g
- Carbohydrates: 2 g
- Protein: 27 g

78. Slow-Cooked Salsa Chicken

Preparation Time: 5 minutes

Cooking Time: 2 hours

Servings: 6

Ingredients:

- 3 pounds boneless, skinless chicken breasts
- 2 cups mild salsa
- 1 cup shredded Mexican Blend cheese

Direction:

1. Place the chicken in your slow cooker and add the mild salsa.
2. Cover with a lid. Cook on "High" for 1 hour and 30 minutes to 2 hours.
3. Preheat your oven to 425°F.
4. Transfer the chicken to a greased baking dish and sprinkle with the Mexican blend cheese.
5. Place in your oven and bake for 15 minutes or until golden brown.
6. Serve and enjoy!

Nutrition:

- Calories: 351
- Fat: 9 g
- Fiber: 1 g
- Carbohydrates: 8 g
- Protein: 54 g

79. Chicken with Mustard Sauce and Bacon

Preparation Time: 10 minutes

Cooking Time: 30 minutes

Servings: 3

Ingredients:

- 2 pounds boneless, skinless chicken breast
- 1/3 cup Dijon mustard
- ¼ teaspoon fine sea salt
- ¼ teaspoon smoked paprika or regular paprika
- 8 medium bacon slices, finely chopped
- 1 small white or red onion, finely chopped
- 1 tablespoon extra-virgin olive oil
- 1 ½ cup homemade low-sodium chicken broth

Directions:

1. In a small bowl, add the Dijon mustard, smoked paprika, fine sea salt, and freshly cracked black pepper. Stir until well combined.
2. Baste the Dijon mustard mixture all over the chicken breast.
3. In a large skillet over medium-high heat, add the bacon and chopped onions and cook until brown and crispy. Transfer to a plate lined with paper towels.
4. Add 1 tablespoon of extra-virgin olive oil to the skillet. Add the chicken and cook for 2 minutes per side. Transfer the chicken to a plate.
5. Pour the chicken broth into the skillet and raise the heat until begins to bubble. Return the cooked bacon and chopped onions to the skillet.
6. Return the chicken to the skillet and reduce the heat. Cover with a lid and allow to simmer for 15 to 20 minutes or until the chicken is thoroughly cooked.
7. Serve and enjoy!

Nutrition:

- Calories: 681
- Fat: 9 g
- Fiber: 2 g
- Carbohydrates: 8 g
- Protein: 74 g

80. Incredibly Delicious Lasagna

Preparation Time: 10 minutes

Cooking Time: 1 hour 30 minutes

Servings: 4

Ingredients:

- 1 pound lean grass-fed ground beef
- 1 (16-ounce) package of lasagna noodles
- 1 cup shredded mozzarella cheese
- 1 onion, finely chopped
- ½ cup mushrooms, finely chopped
- 1 pint ricotta cheese
- ¼ cup Parmesan cheese, finely grated
- 2 eggs
- 1 (28-ounce) jar of spaghetti sauce
- 1 (16-ounce) package of cottage cheese

Directions:

1. Preheat your oven to 350°F.
2. In a large skillet over medium-high heat, add the ground beef and cook until brown.
3. Add the chopped mushrooms and onions. Cook until the mushrooms and onions have softened, stirring occasionally.
4. Stir in the spaghetti sauce and allow it to heat through.
5. In a medium bowl, add the cottage cheese, ricotta cheese, Parmesan grated cheese, and eggs. Stir until well combined.
6. Spread a layer of the meat mixture into a greased baking dish.
7. Layer with lasagna noodles.
8. Spread the cheese mixture over the lasagna noodles and sprinkle with the mozzarella cheese.
9. Add another layer of meat mixture and repeat with all the ingredients. Make sure you have ½ cup of shredded mozzarella cheese left.
10. Cover the baking dish with foil and place it inside your oven. Bake for 45 minutes.
11. Remove the aluminum foil and sprinkle with the remaining ½ cup of shredded mozzarella cheese. Bake for 15 minutes.
12. Remove from your oven and let cool. Serve and enjoy!

Nutrition:

- Calories: 712
- Fat: 31 g
- Fiber: 6 g
- Carbohydrates: 50 g
- Protein: 44 g

81. Kamut Savory Salad

Preparation Time: 10 minutes

Cooking Time: 20 minutes

Servings: 5

Ingredients:

- 1 cup kamut grain, soaked in water overnight, drained
- ¼ cup frozen mixed vegetables
- 1 small carrot, chopped
- ½ cup mixed bell pepper, chopped
- 1 small onion, chopped
- ¼ cup canned or cooked red kidney beans
- 1 teaspoon olive oil
- 3 cups vegetable stock
- Salt to taste
- Pepper to taste
- Spring onion, to garnish
- Parsley, to garnish

Directions:

1. Add kamut and stock into a saucepan. Place the saucepan over medium heat. Cook until tender. Set aside.
2. Place a pan over medium heat. Add oil. When the oil is heated, add onion and sauté until translucent.
3. Add the rest of the ingredients and stir. Heat thoroughly.
4. Sprinkle spring onions and parsley and serve.

Nutrition:

- Calories: 170
- Fat: 8 g
- Fiber: 2 g
- Carbohydrates: 8 g
- Protein: 4 g

82. Beef Satay with Vegetables

Preparation Time: 10 minutes

Cooking Time: 50 minutes

Servings: 4

Ingredients:

- ½ lb. flank steak cut into quarter-inch strips
- 2 teaspoons paste of Thai red curry
- ½ teaspoon fresh ginger ground
- ¼ cup milk from coconuts
- 1 teaspoon monk fruit sweetener granulated
- ¼ cup Natural butter of peanuts
- 2 teaspoons low-sodium soy sauce
- 1 teaspoon lemon juice
- 1 teaspoon extra-virgin olive oil
- 2 cauliflower heads grated
- ¼ teaspoon salt
- ¼ teaspoon freshly ground powder of black pepper
- 1 cup green beans

Directions:

1. Heat an indoor grill in advance.
2. Get a container used for mixing and in it mix the milk from coconuts, natural butter from peanuts, soy sauce, monk fruits sweetener, lemon juice, Thai paste, and fresh ginger that has been ground.
3. Divide the above mixture into two separate containers and in one, add in the flank steak strips.
4. Let the flank steak marinate in the sauce for half an hour.
5. While waiting for foot, the flank steak to marinate, take a non-stick frying skillet and add the olive extra-virgin oil into it.
6. When the oil is nice and hot, add in the grated cauliflower together with black pepper that is freshly ground and salt to season it. Let this cook for 5 minutes.
7. Take the cooked cauliflower from the pan, and in it, add some more olive oil and fry the green beans for 5 minutes until they appear to have a bright green color on them and are not too tender.
8. Take the marinated flanks of steak and grill them on an indoor grill you had heated in advance for about 3 minutes.
9. When ready, serve the grilled flanks of steak with the cooked cauliflower and green beans as well.

Nutrition:

- Calories: 191

- Fat: 9 g
- Fiber: 2 g
- Carbohydrates: 8 g
- Protein: 20 g

83. Parmesan Chicken with Zucchini

Preparation Time: 10 minutes

Cooking Time: 20 minutes

Servings: 6

Ingredients:

- 2 cups minced chicken
- 4 big zucchinis, halved along their length
- 1 cup low-carb tomato basil sauce
- 3 tablespoons extra-virgin olive oil
- ¼ cup Parmesan cheese, grated
- 1 small yellow onion diced
- ¼ cup mozzarella cheese, grated
- 2 garlic cloves minced
- 1 teaspoon basil dried
- ¼ teaspoon salt
- ¼ teaspoon black pepper powder freshly ground

Directions:

1. Heat your oven in advance at 400 °C.
2. Get a large pan used for baking and coat its bottom with the low-carb tomato basil sauce.
3. Get a melon scooper and with care, scoop out the flesh of the zucchini. Take this flesh and blend it gently in a blender.
4. Take a large frying pan and add extra-virgin olive oil to it. Heat the oil over medium heat and when it is hot, add in the diced yellow onion. Let the onion fry for 3 minutes, then add in the minced garlic and cook this for one minute until the garlic is fragrant.
5. Pour in the minced chicken and the blended flesh of zucchini. Season this with the black pepper powder freshly ground and salt. Cover and let this cook for 5 minutes until the chicken is well cooked. Pour out the excess fluid that may remain after the chicken is cooked.
6. Take a little of the sauce and pour it into the cooked chicken stirring so that it covers all the chicken. Let this mixture simmer over medium heat for around 8 minutes.
7. Take the zucchini that has been halved and scooped and place them on a plate. Scoop the minced chicken mixture and place it in the middle of the halved zucchini. Take the stuffed zucchini pieces and place them on the baking dish you prepared earlier.
8. Cover the dish with foil and place it in the oven you had heated in advance. Let them bake in the oven for 25 minutes until the zucchini softens.
9. When the zucchini is soft, take the baking dish from the oven and unwrap the foil. Sprinkle the grated Parmesan and mozzarella cheese at the top. Put back the baking dish in the oven and let it bake until all the cheese melts well.
10. Take it from the oven and serve.

Nutrition:

- Calories: 267
- Fat: 34 g
- Fiber: 2 g
- Carbohydrates: 8 g
- Protein: 46 g

84. Freekeh Salad

Preparation Time: 10 minutes

Cooking Time: 12 minutes

Servings: 2

Ingredients:

- 2 vine tomatoes, chopped or 4 cherry tomatoes, quartered
- Sea salt to taste
- 2 tablespoons olive oil
- Juice of ½ lemon
- Zest of ½ lemon, grated
- A handful fresh cilantro or parsley, chopped
- 1 small cucumber, chopped
- ½ cup corn kernels
- 1 small onion, chopped
- ¾ cup freekeh
- 2 cups water

To Serve

- Hummus or pesto as required
- Avocado slices
- Mini tortillas or wraps, as required

Directions:

1. Add freekeh and water. Place the water over medium heat. When it begins to boil, lower the heat and cover it with a lid. Simmer for 10–12 minutes. Uncover and cook until tender. Drain and set aside.
2. Add lemon juice, oil, lemon zest, salt, and pepper into a small bowl and whisk well.
3. Add the rest of the ingredients, including the freekeh, into a bowl and toss well. Pour dressing on top and toss well. Chill until ready to use.
4. Spread tortillas on your countertop. Place salad on one half of the tortillas. Top with avocado and hummus. Fold the other half over the filling and serve.

Nutrition:

- Calories: 800
- Fat: 8 g
- Fiber: 2 g
- Carbohydrates: 12 g
- Protein: 69 g

85. Kamut, Lentil, and Chickpea Soup

Preparation Time: 10 minutes

Cooking Time: 50 minutes

Servings: 9

Ingredients:

- 1 ½ cup kamut berries, rinsed
- 4 tablespoons olive oil
- 2 cups carrots, finely chopped
- 1 cup celery, thinly sliced
- 4 teaspoons fresh thyme, chopped
- 4 cloves garlic, minced
- 4 bay leaves
- ½ teaspoon pepper powder
- A handful celery leaves, chopped (optional)
- 4 cups boiling water
- 4 cups onion, finely chopped
- 1 ½ cup fresh parsley, chopped
- 2 tablespoons chopped fresh thyme
- 8 cans (14.5 ounces each) chicken broth or use equivalent homemade broth
- 2/3 cup dried lentils, rinsed, soaked in water for 20 minutes
- 2 cans (15 ounces each) chickpeas, rinsed, drained

Directions:

1. Add kamut into a bowl. Cover with boiling water. Let it soak for 30 minutes.
2. Place a soup pot over medium heat. Add oil. When the oil is heated, add onion and herbs and sauté until onions are translucent.
3. Add garlic and sauté until fragrant.
4. Add the rest of the ingredients except chickpeas and stir. Cover and cook until tender.
5. Ladle into soup bowls. Sprinkle celery and serve.

Nutrition:

- Calories: 800
- Fat: 8 g
- Fiber: 2 g
- Carbohydrates: 12 g
- Protein: 69 g

86. Colombian Steak with Onions and Tomatoes

Preparation Time: 10 minutes

Cooking Time: 50 minutes

Servings: 6

Ingredients:

- 1 ½ pound grass-fed sirloin tip steak, sliced thinly
- 1 medium onion, sliced or chopped thinly
- 1 large tomato (or 2 medium tomatoes), sliced or chopped thinly
- 4 teaspoons olive oil, divided
- Garlic powder, to season
- Cumin, to season
- Salt and pepper, to taste
- ¼ cup water

Directions:

1. Season the steak with garlic powder and salt.
2. Place a large skillet over high heat. Add 2 tablespoons of oil and heat. Working in batches, cook the first half of the steak for about 1 minute. Stir halfway to cook evenly. Once cooked, transfer to a plate. Do this step to the remaining batch and then set aside.
3. Reduce the heat to medium. Using the same pan, heat oil and sauté the onions for 2 minutes. Add the tomatoes and season with cumin, salt, and pepper. Reduce the heat to medium-low.
4. Add about a ¼ cup of water and let simmer for a few minutes to reduce the liquid volume. Add more water if needed and adjust the taste accordingly.
5. Return the steak to the skillet with its drippings. Mix well before removing the pan from the heat.
6. Serve with rice or a fried egg on top.

Nutrition:

- Calories: 378
- Fat: 8 g
- Fiber: 2 g
- Carbohydrates: 8 g
- Protein: 6 g

87. Maple Walnut-Glazed Black-Eyed Peas with Collard Greens

Preparation Time: 10 minutes
Cooking Time: 30 minutes
Servings: 3

Ingredients:

For the Maple-Walnut Glaze

- ¾ cup water
- ½ cup walnuts, chopped
- ½ tablespoon Tamari sauce
- 2 tablespoons sugar-free maple syrup
- 1 teaspoon arrowroot starch flour
- Dash of nutmeg
- ½ teaspoon ground mustard
- 1/8 teaspoon ground ginger
- 1/8 teaspoon ground cinnamon
- 1/8 teaspoon ground cloves

For the Black-Eyed Peas and Collard Greens

- 4 cups cooked black-eyed peas
- 1 large bunch fresh collard greens, cleaned, stems removed, and chopped
- ¼ cup water (plus more)

Directions:

1. For the maple-walnut glaze, put all ingredients in a blender in this order: water, walnuts, tamari, maple syrup, starch and spices. Blend starting at the lowest setting and gradually adjust to the highest. Blend on high for about 40 seconds. Set aside.
2. For the peas and collards, place a 5-quart sauté pan over medium-high heat and add water. Put the collards and steam-sauté until tender, about 10 minutes. You can also adjust the doneness according to your preference.
3. Add the glaze to the greens and continue to cook on medium-high for about 2 minutes. Stir frequently.
4. Add the peas. Continue to cook and stir another minute. Serve immediately.

Nutrition:

- Calories: 233
- Fat: 8 g
- Fiber: 2 g
- Carbohydrates: 8 g
- Protein: 13 g

CHAPTER 13.

—·——·——❦——·——·—

DESSERT RECIPES: 12 RECIPES

88. Coconut Custard Pie

Preparation Time: 10 minutes

Cooking Time: 50 minutes

Servings: 8

Ingredients:

- 1 cup heavy whipping cream
- ¾ cup powdered Erythritol-based sweetener
- ½ cup full-fat coconut Milk
- 4 large eggs
- ½ stick (¼ cup) cooled, unsalted, melted butter
- 1¼ cups unsweetened shredded coconut
- 3 tablespoons coconut flour
- ½ teaspoon baking powder
- ½ teaspoon vanilla extract
- ¼ teaspoon salt

Directions:

1. Heat the oven to 350°F and grease a 9-inch ceramic pie pan or glass.
2. Place the melted butter, eggs, coconut milk, sweetener, and cream in a blender. Blend well.
3. Add the vanilla extract, baking powder, salt, coconut flour, and a cup of shredded coconut. Continue blending.
4. Empty the mixture into the pie pan and sprinkle with the rest of the shredded coconut. Bake for 40–50 minutes and stop when the center is jiggly but the sides are set.
5. Take out of the oven and allow it to cool for 30 minutes. Place in the refrigerator and let it rest for 2 hours before cutting it.

Nutrition:

- **Fat:** 29.5 g
- Carbohydrates: 6.7 g
- Protein: 5.3 g
- Calories: 317

89. Dairy-Free Fruit Tarts

Preparation Time: 15 minutes

Cooking Time: 15 minutes

Servings: 2

Ingredients:

- 1 cup coconut whipped cream
- ½ easy shortbread crust (dairy-free option)
- Fresh mint sprigs
- ½ cup mixed fresh berries

Directions:

1. Grease two 4" pans with detachable bottoms. Pour the shortbread mixture into the pans and firmly press into the edges and bottom of each pan. Cook for 15 minutes.
2. Loosen the crust carefully to remove it from the pan.
3. Distribute the whipped cream between the tarts and evenly spread it to the sides. Refrigerate for 1–2 hours to make it firm.
4. Use the berries and sprig of mint to garnish each of the tarts.

Nutrition:

- **Fats:** 28.9 g
- Carbohydrates: 8.3 g
- Protein: 5.8 g
- Calories: 306

90. Strawberry Rhubarb Crisp

Preparation Time: 10 minutes

Cooking Time: 30 minutes

Servings: 2

Ingredients:

Topping Ingredients

- 1 tablespoon unsweetened shredded coconut
- 2 ½ tablespoons blanched almond flour
- 1 ½ teaspoon finely chopped pecans
- 1 tablespoon granulated Erythritol-based sweetener
- Pinch of salt
- 2 teaspoons melted unsalted butter
- ¼ teaspoon ground cinnamon

Filling Ingredients

- 1/3 cup sliced fresh strawberries
- ½ cup chopped fresh rhubarb
- 1/16 teaspoon xanthan gum
- 1 tablespoon granulated Erythritol-based sweetener

Directions:

1. Preparing the Topping Ingredients:
2. Heat the oven to 300°F and line a baking sheet with parchment paper.
3. Whisk the cinnamon, pecans, salt, sweetener, coconut, and almond flour in a medium bowl. Add the melted butter into the mixture and stir until the resulting mixture appears like coarse crumbs.
4. Place on the coated baking sheet and firmly press down to make it flat. Bake for and 15 minutes then allow it to cool.
5. Preparing the Filling and Assembling Ingredients:
6. Heat the oven to 400°F.
7. Add all the filling ingredients into a medium bowl and make sure that you thoroughly mix them. Place into an 8-ounce ramekin and cover with foil. Place in the oven to bake for 10–15 minutes.

Nutrition:

- Calories: 135
- **Fats:** 11.5 g
- Protein: 2.6 g

91. Raspberry Fool

Preparation Time: 15 minutes

Cooking Time: 0 minute

Servings: 4

Ingredients:

- 2–4 tablespoons powdered and divided Erythritol-based sweetener
- 1 cup thawed frozen raspberries
- Fresh berries, for garnish
- 1 cup whipped cream

Directions:

1. Process 2 tablespoons of sweetener and berries in a food processor or blender until smooth. Fold in the raspberry puree into the whipped cream, leaving some streaks.
2. Pour the mixture into four dessert cups. Garnish with the berries.

Nutrition:

- **Fats:** 20.1 g
- Carbohydrates: 5.2 g
- Protein: 1.7 g
- Fiber: 1 g

92. Raspberry Chia Pudding

Preparation Time: 10 minutes

Cooking Time: 0 minute

Servings: 2

Ingredients:

- 4 tablespoons chia seeds
- ½ cup raspberries
- 1 cup coconut milk

Directions:

1. Pour the milk and raspberries into a blender. Pulse until smooth. Pour into the jars.
2. Fold in the chia seeds and stir. Secure the lid and shake. Store in the fridge for at least 3 hours before serving.

Nutrition:

- Protein: 38.8
- Total Fats: 28.3 g
- Calories: 408

93. Squash Pudding

Preparation Time: 5 minutes

Cooking Time: 0 minute

Servings: 1

Ingredients:

- ½ cup water
- 2 cups squash
- 7 dates, pitted
- 2 tablespoons coconut oil, virgin
- 2 tablespoons peanut butter
- 1 small ginger cube
- ½ vanilla bean pod, scraped
- 1 ½ tablespoon cloves

Directions:

1. Pour water into a food processor and then all other ingredients. Process until a creamy texture.
2. Serve and enjoy!

Nutrition:

- Calories: 703
- Protein: 11 g
- Sugar: 45 g
- **Fiber:** 15 g

94. Strawberries with Coconut Whip

Preparation Time: 10 minutes

Cooking Time: 0 minute

Servings: 4

Ingredients:

- 4 cups strawberries or other favorite berries
- 2 cans refrigerated coconut cream
- 1 ounce 70% or darker unsweetened chopped dark chocolate

Directions:

1. Remove the solidified cream from the can of milk and set it aside for another time, saving the liquid. Pour it into a mixing container and whip it with a hand mixer until it forms stiff peaks (approximately five minutes).
2. Slice the berries and portion them into four dishes. Serve with a dollop of the cream. Garnish with the chopped chocolate and a few berries. Serve.

Nutrition:

- Net Carbohydrates: 10 g
- Protein: 4 g
- Calories: 342

95. Almond Blackberry Chia Pudding

Preparation Time: 15 minutes

Cooking Time: 0 minute

Servings: 2

Ingredients:

- ¼ cup chia seeds
- Drizzle raw honey
- 2 tablespoons sliced almonds
- 1 ½ cup vanilla almond milk
- 6 ounce fresh blackberries

Directions:

1. Rinse and add the berries into a dish. Crush with a fork until creamy. Pour in the raw honey, milk, and chia seeds. Stir well. Refrigerate for several hours or overnight for the most delicious results.
2. Sprinkle with the almonds and several blackberries. Serve any time.

Nutrition:

- Net Carbohydrates: 1 g
- Protein: 2 g
- Calories: 109

96. Choco Mug Brownie

Preparation Time: 10 minutes

Cooking Time: 30 seconds

Servings: 1

Ingredients:

- 1 tablespoon cocoa powder
- ½ teaspoon baking powder
- 1 scoop chocolate protein powder
- ¼ cup almond milk

Directions:

1. Prepare a mug using protein powder, cocoa, and baking powder. Pour the milk into the mug and stir. Microwave for about 30 seconds and serve.

Nutrition:

- Protein: 12.4 g
- Total Fats: 15.8 g
- Calories: 207

97. Chocolate Mousse

Preparation Time: 1 hour

Cooking Time: 0 minute

Servings: 2

Ingredients:

- 4 tablespoons butter
- 4 tablespoons cream cheese
- 1 ½ tablespoon heavy whipping cream
- 1 tablespoon swerve or another natural sweetener
- 1 tablespoon unsweetened cocoa powder

Directions:

1. Remove the butter and cream cheese from the fridge for about 30 minutes before it is time to prepare them so that they are at room temperature. Chill a bowl and whisk the cream. Place back in the refrigerator for now.
2. Use a hand mixer to combine the sweetener, cream cheese, cocoa powder, and butter until well mixed. Remove the refrigerated cream and fold it into the chocolate mixture using a rubber scraper.
3. Portion it into two dessert bowls and chill for one hour.

Nutrition:

- Protein: 4 g
- Total Fats: 50 g
- Calories: 460

98. Chocolate Muffins

Preparation Time: 20 minutes

Cooking Time: 5 minutes

Servings: 6

Ingredients:

- ½ cup coconut oil
- ½ cup peanut butter
- Liquid stevia granulated sweetener (to your liking)

Directions:

1. Prepare the tin of choice with a spritz of oil. Combine the oil and peanut butter together on the stovetop or microwave. Melt and add the sweetener. Scoop into the tins or loaf pan and freeze.
2. You can serve with a drizzle of melted chocolate—but remember to count the carbs.

Nutrition:

- Protein: 7 g
- Total Fats: 14 g
- Calories: 193

99. Cannoli Dessert Dip

Preparation Time: 10 minutes

Cooking Time: 10 minutes

Servings: 8

Ingredients:

- ¾ cup (6 ounces) softened cream cheese
- 1 cup whole-milk ricotta cheese at room temperature
- ½ teaspoon Vanilla extract
- ¾ cup powdered Erythritol-based sweetener, plus an additional amount for sprinkling
- 1/3 cup sugarless chocolate chips
- ½ cup heavy whipping cream

Directions:

1. Blend the vanilla extract, sweetener, cream cheese, and ricotta in a food processor or blender until smooth.
2. Whisk in the cream using an electric mixer in a medium bowl until it holds solid peaks. Carefully fold in the chocolate chips and the ricotta mixture and save some for later to sprinkle on top.

Nutrition:

- Calories: 219
- **Fats:** 17.9 g
- Carbohydrates: 5.6 g
- Protein: 5.7 g

CONCLUSION

If you are a woman over the age of 50, intermittent fasting may be beneficial to you. However, it is not a cure-all. You need to consult your doctor before embarking on any kind of fast. It is not recommended for women with a history of breast cancer, diabetes, or liver disease. Most women over the age of 50 who try intermittent fasting report that they feel better throughout the day. This reinforces the idea that fasts can be part of our lives as we age, but a doctor must first be consulted before attempting one.

Several fasts can improve your health. While long fasts can get very difficult, some short fasts can be just as effective at improving your health. In general, it is essential to reduce long fasts if you have trouble with them. If you want to experiment with shorter fasts, try eating less and sleeping more for two days, and then eating normally the next two days. Fasting can be beneficial when used in a short cycle.

There is no specific time frame that should be used for fasting when trying to improve health because it all depends on the individual's circumstances and goals for the fast. For some people, intermittent fasting or longer fasts are useful if they are trying to lose weight, while others use them to manage their diabetes or heart disease. This lifestyle is perfect for women over the age of 50. It allows women to reap the benefits of moderate-length fasts without giving their bodies time to adapt to stress from food deprivation. It can also help women who have trouble sleeping during long fasts since it does not require as much sleep time every night. This eating pattern allows people to have more time between meals, enabling them to avoid snacking, which can lead to gaining weight if eaten frequently while fasting.

Intermittent fasting is a popular weight-loss technique that has been making headlines lately. It involves limiting eating to a specific period of time each day and then allowing yourself to eat normally for the remainder of the day.

It is not a diet but rather a way to increase your metabolism and lose weight. It works by resetting your body's clock to burn fat at a higher rate and increase your metabolic rate (the rate at which your body uses energy and processes toxins).

The best way to start intermittent fasting is by establishing reliable eating windows or time frames during which you allow yourself to eat normally. This gives your body time to switch from being in "fasting" mode, burning fat at a higher rate, to the "fed" way, where it burns sugar and carbs instead. Your weight loss will begin after you've achieved this goal.

However, if you find that you can't stop eating after a few hours despite having set an eating window for yourself, you may be suffering from intermittent fasting.

Prone to heartburn and indigestion, women over the age of 50 seem to suffer from these maladies frequently. Here are some things you can try to avoid this type of discomfort:

- The most effective way to avoid heartburn and indigestion is to eat when your stomach is empty. You must eat slowly and chew your food thoroughly. If you have trouble with chewing, have a glass of water nearby so you can take small sips while you're eating. Sipping will help keep your food moving through the digestive system.

- If you are eating with other people, everyone must sit down at the table simultaneously. Try to avoid eating in front of a television or a computer monitor while seated on the couch or your bed. People who eat in these ways tend to eat less than those who sit down at the table and talk with others around them at the table.

- If you are having heartburn problems or indigestion, ask your doctor about prescription meds for heartburn or indigestion. These drugs are much better than over-the-counter products that can cause more harm than good.

- Occasional fasts are another option you may want to consider if you have frequent problems with heartburn and indigestion. However, if you do fast every day, make sure that you don't skip meals altogether because this can lead to health complications such as hypoglycemia or low blood sugar.

CPSIA information can be obtained
at www.ICGtesting.com
Printed in the USA
BVHW061031220621
610126BV00006B/713